国際学会 English
スピーキング・エクササイズ
口演・発表・応答 　*C.S.Langham*（日本大学特任教授）著

ENGLISH FOR
ORAL
PRESENTATIONS
SPEAKING
EXERCISES

医歯薬出版株式会社

■音声データのダウンロードとご利用について

- 本書中の の番号は音声データのトラックナンバーを示しています.
- 音声データは下記の URL または QR コードから無料でダウンロードすることができます.

  https://www.ishiyaku.co.jp/ebooks/433680/

<注意事項>

- 再生には MP3 形式の音声データを再生できるプレイヤーが必要です.
- お客様がご負担になる通信料金について十分にご理解のうえご利用をお願いします.
- 音声データを無断で複製・公に上映・公衆送信（送信可能化を含む）・翻訳・翻案することは法律により禁止されています.

<お問合せ先>

  https://www.ishiyaku.co.jp/ebooks/inquiry/

This book is originally published in Japanese
under the title of :

KOKUSAI GAKKAI INGURISSHU SUPIKINGU EKUSASAIZU
(English for Oral Presentations : Speaking Exercises)

C. S. Langham
  Professor at Nihon University School of Dentistry

© 2023 1st ed.

ISHIYAKU PUBLISHERS, INC.
  7-10, Honkomagome 1 chome, Bunkyo-ku,
  Tokyo 113-8612, Japan

Introduction

Oral presentations have become one of the main ways of transmitting research results and an essential tool for professionals in a variety of fields. They are also important for graduate students and, to a lesser extent, undergraduates.

This book aims at meeting the needs of presenters who are non-native speakers of English. It is based on the author's experience of teaching presentation skills at universities and institutes in Japan over a period of twenty five years. During that time, I have noted a significant improvement in presentations given by Japanese presenters, but problems remain and, in my opinion, these are not simply matters of grammar or pronunciation. In fact, they are far more serious. For example, many presentations lack a clear framework, conform more to the rules of a written paper than an oral presentation, and do not distinguish between foreground and background.

In this book, I focus on ways of overcoming these and other problems. My approach is a linguistic one and I concentrate on the English you need to present your data. There are many example sentences and vocabulary items that you can use to improve your presentation and make your data more convincing. This book comes with an audio file and has exercises that will help you to improve your speaking and listening ability, and also remember the key sentences and vocabulary presented here. It has four complete example introductions and three complete example conclusions. There are several quick guides that provide easy access to the language you need. Additionally, there is one interview with an experienced presenter and ten thought-provoking topics on presentations that introduce useful techniques.

You can use this book as a reference when you are preparing your next presentation and also as a textbook for improving your speaking and listening skills.

A c k n o w l e d g m e n t s

I wish to thank the following people who kindly allowed me access to their presentations, data and graphics. Professor A. R. Cools, Department of Psychoneuropharmacology, Nijmegen University, the Netherlands. Professor J. L. Waddington, Department of Molecular and Cellular Therapeutics, Royal College of Surgeons in Ireland. Dr. Mathew Brett, the MRC-Cognition and Brain Sciences Unit, Cambridge University, Cambridge, England. Dr. Patrick Micke, the Cancer Center, Karolinska, Stockholm, Sweden. Dr. Amar Gandavadi, Birmingham University, School of Health Sciences, Physiotherapy, University of Birmingham, Edgbaston, Birmingham, England. Dr. Toshiyuki Kanamori, Institute of Advanced Industrial Science and Technology, Japan. I also wish to acknowledge my friend and colleague, Brian Purdue of Tsukuba University, with whom over the years I have had many valuable discussions concerning presentation techniques. Thanks are also due to Dan Waldhoff for his help with recording. Finally, I should also like to thank Michael Jones for his useful comments on the manuscript.

Clive Langham
Nihon University
School of Dentistry
Ochanomizu, Tokyo
February 1st, 2010

CONTENTS

Presentation Topics

Presentation Topics

In this book, there are ten presentation topics that introduce suggestions for improving your presentation skills. Before reading the text, listen to the topic on the audio file several times. If you want extra listening practice, transcribe the topic from the audio file and then check your version against the text. I hope you will find these topics interesting and that they will help you to give better presentations in the future.

Presentation Techniques

In this book, there is a discussion about presentation techniques. I have included it here, because I think the ideas and techniques discussed will be useful for you. It also provides listening practice. The best way to approach this discussion is to listen to the audio file several times and complete the listening exercises 1 ~10. Then, after you have checked your answers, listen to the audio file again and read the script. If there are any techniques or ideas that interest you, think about using them in your next presentation.

Part 1

Starting your presentation

I n part 1 of this book, I want to consider effective ways of starting a presentation.

1 You need a framework

I would like to start by considering part of a discussion on presentation skills with Dr. Alexander Cools that was recorded at Nihon University School of Dentistry on October 10th, 2008.

L : I'm interested in ways of starting presentations. I'd like to ask you about the best way to start.

C : I think you need a framework that shows where you will go in the presentation.

L : Do you mean some kind of overview?

C : Yes, that's correct.

L : Do you think it is possible to start a presentation without a framework or overview?

C : No, I don't. I think you couldn't make a bigger mistake.

L : What about if it is a closed meeting? One where everyone is working in the same field and known to each other.

C : You have to remember that no two specialists are the same. Starting without at least some kind of framework would be like going into a new area without a map.

L = C.S.Langham   C = Dr.Alexander Cools

The following is an analysis of the key points made in the above discussion on presentation skills.

1. I think you need a <u>framework</u> that shows <u>where you will go in the presentation</u>.

The first word I want to focus on in the above sentence is *framework*. It refers to an outline or overview of the presentation which is often in the form of a list of contents. For most presenters, this is the second slide in their presentation and comes after a slide showing the presentation title, as well as the presenter's name and affiliation. The phrase, *where you will go in the presentation*, is also important, since it shows how a framework will indicate the structure and direction of your talk. In some presentations I see, presenters refer to their contents slide several times during their presentation. This is to show where they are now, where they have been and where they are going. Doing this will help the audience to follow the presentation.

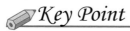

Key Point

●これから何について話そうとしているか，まずその枠組みを示す.

2. You have to remember that <u>no two specialists are the same.</u>

Later in our discussion, I asked if a framework or outline is always necessary. I was thinking here of sessions that consist of small groups of specialists in the same field who meet frequently and are very familiar with each other's research work. Dr. Cools answered my question by saying, *no two specialists are the same*. By this, I think he meant that within the same group there will be people with different levels of knowledge and expertise who approach the same subject from different angles and, as such, a framework as part of your introduction is essential. I think this point is something that we need to keep in mind when starting our presentations.

Key Point

●同じ分野の専門家や同じような研究をしているような人たちの集まりでも，知識レベルや視点はさまざまなので，話の枠組みを示すことを忘れてはならない.

3. Starting without at least <u>some kind of framework</u> would be like <u>going into a new area without a map.</u>

His final comment on starting a presentation is also interesting. Here he stated quite clearly the need for a framework. The key word is *map*. If you do not provide a framework, the audience has no map and, consequently, will find it difficult to follow your presentation. I believe that we need to give our audience a map that will guide them through our presentation.

Key Point

●話の枠組みを示さずに話し始めることは，地図をもたずに見知らぬ土地に行かせるようなもので,聴衆は話の内容についていくのが難しくなる.

2 Example introduction 1

I n the rest of this part, I will give you examples of useful language you can use to create a map for your audience that will help them to follow your presentation.

I'm going to introduce four examples of how to start a presentation. For each of the example introductions, first, do the listening exercises. Then, read the key sentences and explanations that follow them.

Listening 1

Listen to example introduction 1 and answer questions 1 and 2.

1. What is the main topic of the presentation?
   a. new products
   b. side effects
   c. tooth and gum sensitivity
   d. bleaching

2. How many parts does the presentation have?
   a. 1
   b. 2
   c. 3
   d. 4

Listening 2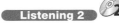

Now listen to the introduction again. Match the words and phrases in 1~6 with those in a~f.

1. Today, I'd like to talk about	a. two new products
2. First, I'll give a brief introduction to	b. our recent case study
3. Next, I'd like to describe	c. possible side effects
4. I'll focus on	d. bleaching
5. In part three, I'm going to look at	e. safe treatment
6. I'll give some suggestions for	f. whitening techniques

Listening 3

Listen again and complete the sentences. Each space has one word only.

Thank you Chairperson. Good morning, everyone. Today, I'd like to _____ _____ bleaching. My presentation is in four parts. First, I'll _____ a brief introduction to whitening techniques. Next, _____ _____ to describe our recent case study. _____ _____ on two new products. These are wraps and strips. In part three, I'm going to _____ _____ possible side effects, such as tooth and gum sensitivity. Finally, I'll _____ some suggestions for safe treatment. Let me _____ _____ whitening techniques.

Listening 4

Listen again. Look at the script and check your answers.

Thank you, Chairperson. Good morning, everyone. Today, I'd like to talk about bleaching. My presentation is in four parts. First, I'll give a brief introduction to whitening techniques. Next, I'd like to describe our recent case study. I'll focus on two new products. These are wraps and strips. In part three, I'm going to look at possible side effects, such as tooth and gum sensitivity. Finally, I'll give some suggestions for safe treatment. Let me start with whitening techniques.

Answers
Listening 1 1-d, 2-d
Listening 2 1-d, 2-f, 3-b, 4-a, 5-c, 6-e
Listening 3 talk about, give, I'd like, I'll focus, look at, give, start with

5

Example introduction 1
Key Sentences

Below, you can see the title of the presentation and the contents slide.

A Clinical Evaluation of Bleaching
Using Whitening Wraps and Strips

Contents
1. Whitening techniques
2. Case study using two products:
   wraps and strips
3. Possible side effects
4. Suggestions for safe treatment

---

1. Good morning, everyone. Today, I'd like to talk about bleaching.

As you can see, the title of the presentation is simple (*A Clinical Evaluation of Bleaching Using Whitening Wraps and Strips*). The presenter does not read the title from the slide. Instead, he starts by introducing the main subject of the presentation, which is bleaching. He introduces the topic of the presentation with the sentence, *I'd like to talk about + topic.*

Key Point

●タイトルは読まずに主テーマを紹介する．その際，'I'd like to talk about' というフレーズが有効である．

2. My presentation is in four parts.

The speaker then starts to build up a map of the presentation by stating the number of parts.

The following sentences can also be used to do this.

- *My presentation has four parts.*
- *I'd like to divide my presentation into four parts.*
- *My presentation consists of four parts.*

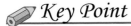 ## Key Point

●講演の内容がいくつのパートから構成されているかを示す.

3. First, I'll give a brief introduction to whitening techniques.

Each of the parts of the overview is introduced in a simple way. In this case, the presenter uses the sentence, *first, I'll + give a brief introduction to + topic.* In this situation, you can also use the following verbs: *I'm going to = I am going to, I'd like to = I would like to,* and *I want to.*

The presenter uses the phrase *give a brief introduction to + topic.*

Here are some other examples of how the word *give* is commonly used in scientific presentations.

- *I want to <u>give an overview of</u> the main advantages of the new system.*
- *I'm going to <u>give an outline of</u> recent developments in this field.*
- *I'd like to <u>give a summary of</u> the results from our recent experiments.*

For more examples using the word *give*, see Quick Guide 2. Starting your presentation – Key Vocabulary: Page 32, No. 2.

Key Point

●全体の構成を示した後, まず最初に何について話すのかを簡単に紹介する. 'First, I'll + give a brief introduction to + topic.' というフレーズが有効である.

4. Next, I'd like to describe our recent case study. I'll focus on two new products. These are wraps and strips.

The second part of the overview is introduced with the word *next*. This is followed by *I'd like to describe + topic*.

The verb *describe* can also be used in the following ways.

- *I'd like to <u>describe</u> a recent case study.*
- *I want to <u>describe</u> a new method.*
- *I'm going to <u>describe</u> some possible applications.*
- *I'll <u>describe</u> the experimental setup.*

For more examples using the word *describe*, see Quick Guide 2. Starting your presentation – Key Vocabulary: Page 34, No. 13.

Also, note that the presenter gives an example of two new products using the verb *focus on + topic*.

Focus on can also be used in the following ways.

- *I'll <u>focus on</u> two new products.*
- *In part two, I'm going to <u>focus on</u> possible applications.*
- *I'd like to <u>focus on</u> recent modifications to the system.*
- *My main <u>focus</u> today in this presentation will be on animal models.*
  (In this case, focus is used as a noun)

For more examples using *focus on*, see Quick Guide 2. Starting your presentation – Key Vocabulary: Page 34, No. 12.

🖊 *Key Point*

- 'next' を使って，次に何について話すのかを示す．その際，'describe' や 'focus on' を使用すると有効である．

5. In part three, I'm going to look at possible side effects, such as tooth and gum sensitivity.

The presenter uses the phrase *in part three* to indicate the next section. It is also possible to say *in the third part*.

The verb *look at* has a wide range of meanings and here means *consider*. The presenter gives an example of possible side effects by using the phrase *such as + example*.

Here are some more examples using the verb *look at*.

• *In part two, I'm going to look at the symptoms of the disease.*
• *I'm also going to look at several different types of treatment.*
• *In the third part, I want to look at side effects and how to limit them.*

For more examples using *look at*, see Quick Guide 2. Starting your presentation – Key Vocabulary:Page 33, No. 8.

Key Point

● その次の話を説明するときは 'in part three' や 'in the third part' を使う. その際に使う動詞として 'look at' は幅広く使える.

6. Finally, I'll give some suggestions for safe treatment.

The last section in the introduction is indicated by the word *finally*. It is also possible to say *lastly*, and *in the last / final section*.

Key Point

● 最後の内容を紹介するときは, 'finally' や 'lastly' を使う.

7. Let me start with whitening techniques.

The presenter finishes the introduction with the above sentence and in this way moves on to part one of the presentation. This is a smooth transition from the last part of the introduction to part one of the main body, using the phrase *Let me start with + topic*.

Key Point

● 本題に移るときは 'Let me start with + topic' を使う.

3 Example introduction 2

T he following is part of a presentation entitled Functional imaging of the human brain given at Nihon University School of Dentistry by Dr. Mathew Brett of the MRC-Cognition and Brain Sciences Unit, Cambridge University.

Listening 1

Listen to this introduction and answer questions 1 and 2.

1. What is the topic of the presentation? Choose one from a∼d below.
    a. PET (positron emission tomography)
    b. FMRI (functional magnetic resonance imaging)
    c. Functional brain imaging
    d. How the brain works

2. How many sections are there?
    Circle one: 1, 2, 3, 4,

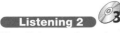

Listening 2

Now listen again and complete sentences 1~7.

1. Today, I'm going to _____ _____ functional brain imaging.
2. Just briefly, before I start, _____ _____ _____ _____ some of the people who have been involved in these slides, as well as this work.
3. So today, I'm going to _____ _____ _____ _____ function-al brain imaging.
4. Firstly, I'm going to _____ what functional brain imaging is.
5. Then, in the next section, I'm going to _____ the question: What can it tell you?
6. After that, I'm going to _____ _____ _____ _____ about how two of the main techniques work - which are PET and FMRI.
7. Finally, I'm going to _____ _____ _____ of where brain imag-ing has been successful in telling us new things about how the brain works.

Listening 3

Listen again. Look at the script and check your answers.

Thank you very much for your kind introduction. Today, I'm going to talk about functional brain imaging. Just briefly, before I start, I'd like to thank some of the people who have been involved in these slides, as well as this work (The presenter shows a slide with a list of names and gives a short explanation). So today, I'm going to give an overview of functional brain imaging. Firstly, I'm going to discuss what functional brain imag-ing is. Then, in the next section, I'm going to ask the question: What can it tell you? - which is how the brain works and, therefore, what it can be used for. After that, I'm going to go into some detail about how two of the main techniques work - which are PET and FMRI. Finally, I'm going to discuss some examples of where brain imaging has been successful in telling us new things about how the brain works.

Answers

Listening 1 1-c, 2-4

Listening 2 1.talk about, 2.I'd like to thank, 3.give an overview of, 4.discuss, 5.ask, 6.go into some detail, 7.discuss some examples

Example introduction 2
Key Sentences

1. Today, I'm going to talk about functional brain imaging.

The presenter starts by introducing the topic of the presentation, and not by reading the title. It's not necessary to read the title because it is on the first slide, in the conference handbook and has just been announced by the Chairperson. To introduce the topic, the presenter uses the sentence, *Today, I'm going to talk about functional brain imaging*. The pattern is *talk about + topic* which is the same sentence pattern as used in example introduction 1 on page 6.

Key Point

● ここでも，タイトルは読まずに'talk about + topic' を使って主テーマを紹介している．

2. Just briefly, before I start, I'd like to thank some of the people who have been involved in these slides as well as this work.

Most presenters acknowledge their coworkers at the end of their presentation. In this case, however, the presenter includes this information at the start of the presentation. Personally, I think it is more appropriate to do this at the end of the presentation, but both are possible. Notice that the presenter uses the phrase *I'd like to thank*, when acknowledging coworkers. Here are some more examples of how to acknowledge people.

- *I'd like to thank the following people* (+ list of names).
- *I'd like to acknowledge the people who have worked with us on this project* (+ list of names).

For more examples of how to acknowledge people , see Quick Guide 3. Starting your presentation – Key Sentences: Page 85, No. 5.

Key Point

● 謝辞は最後に述べたほうが効果的であるが，最初に言ってしまってもよい．

3. So today, I'm going to give an overview of functional brain imaging.

After the acknowledgment, the presenter repeats the theme of the presentation. Notice the use of the phrase, *give an overview of + topic*.

For more examples using the word *give*, see Quick Guide 2. Starting your presentation – Key Vocabulary: Page 32, No. 2.

Key Point

● 'give an overview of + topic' のフレーズでテーマを紹介している.

4. Firstly, I'm going to discuss what functional brain imaging is.

The presenter introduces part one of the presentation using the word *firstly* and then uses, *I'm going to discuss + topic*. In this case, he uses the phrase, *what functional brain imaging is*. It would also be possible to say, *I'm going to discuss functional brain imaging*.

Key Point

● 'firstly' 'I'm going to discuss + topic' で最初の話題を紹介している.

5. Then, in the next section, I'm going to ask the question: What can it tell you? - which is how the brain works and, therefore, what it can be used for.

He introduces part two of the introduction with the word, *then*. It would also be possible to use *next*. Note that he uses a question to attract the attention of the audience. *What can it tell you?* He then answers the question by giving two examples of what the technique can tell us.

For more examples of how to use questions in your presentation see, Using questions in the main body, on page 60.

Key Point

● 'then' を使って次の話題を紹介する一方で, 聴衆の関心を引くために疑問形を使っている.

6. After that, I'm going to go into some detail about how two of the main techniques work - which are PET and FMRI.

The next section is introduced with the phrase *after that*. He then uses the phrase, *I'm going to go into some detail about + topic*. The phrase, *go into some detail*, means to explain in detail. For example: *I'm going to explain in detail about + topic*.

✏️ *Key Point*

●その次の話題の紹介には 'after that' と 'I'm going to go into some detail about + topic' を使っている.

7. Finally, I'm going to discuss some examples of where brain imaging has been successful in telling us new things about how the brain works.

The last section of the introduction is introduced with the word *finally*. It would also be possible to say *lastly* or *in the last / final section*. The presenter also uses the sentence, *I'm going to discuss + topic*.

For more examples using the word *discuss*, see Quick Guide 2. Starting your presentation – Key Vocabulary: Page 34, No. 10.

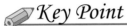

Key Point

●最後の話題の紹介には 'finally' と 'I'm going to discuss + topic' を使っている.

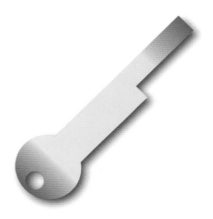

4 Example introduction 3 (Part 1)

This is part of a presentation given by Dr. Patrick Micke entitled Exploring the tumor environment: Gene expression profiling of cancer associated fibroblasts. Dr. Micke works at the Cancer Center, Karolinska, Stockholm, Sweden. Please note that he is an invited speaker.

Listening 1

Listen and complete these notes by matching the words and phrases in 1~5 with those in a~e.

1. job_____
2. previously worked in_____
3. currently doing research at_____
4. wants to give_____
5. and present_____

a. our ongoing work
b. a brief introduction to our research field
c. the Cancer Center Karolinska
d. the Department of Oncology
e. medical doctor

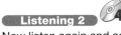

Listening 2

Now listen again and complete sentences 1~5.

1. _____ _____ _____ _____ by saying how pleased I am to be able to speak to you today.
2. It is indeed a great _____ and an _____ to be here.
3. As you probably know, I am a medical doctor and I _____ _____several years as a physician in the Department of Oncology.
4. Currently, I am _____ _____ at the Cancer Center, Karolinska.
5. I would like to _____ _____ _____ _____ to our research field and _____ our ongoing work.

Listening 3

Now listen again and check your answers.

Thank you very much for your kind introduction. I'd like to start by saying how pleased I am to be able to speak to you today. It is indeed a great pleasure and an honor to be here. As you probably know, I am a medical doctor and I worked for several years as a physician in the Department of Oncology. Currently, I am doing research at the Cancer Center Karolinska in the group of Professor Arne Ostman in Stockholm. I would like to give a brief introduction to our research field and present our ongoing work.

Answers

Listening 1 1-e, 2-d, 3-c, 4-b, 5-a
Listening 2 1.I'd like to start, 2.pleasure, honor, 3.worked for, 4.doing research, 5.give a brief introduction, present

**1. I'd like to start by saying how pleased I am to be able
to speak to you today. It is indeed a great pleasure
and an honor to be here.**

As the presenter is an invited speaker, he makes some general remarks
before starting his presentation. These remarks are quite formal.

Here are several examples that can be used if you are an invited speaker.
However, please note these sentences are too formal for presentations
where you are one of a number of presenters speaking in a regular session.
They should only be used if you are an invited speaker.

- *It's a great honor to be able to speak to you today.*
- *It gives me great pleasure to speak here today.*
- *I'm very pleased to have the opportunity to present my research at
this conference.*
- *I'm delighted to have this chance to speak to you today.*
- *I would like to express my sincere thanks to Dr. Jones and the orga-
nizing committee for inviting me to speak here.*

Key Point

● ゲストとしてただ1人講演をする場合は，上記のフレーズを使って自分
の気持ちを表現してよい.

2. I am a medical doctor and I worked for several years as a physician in the Department of Oncology. Currently, I am doing research at the Cancer Center Karolinska in the group of Professor Arne Ostman in Stockholm.

Sometimes, particularly if you are an invited speaker, it is useful to give the audience some information about your field, research interests, and place of work. This will help them to understand who you are and what you are doing. It will also probably help them to follow your presentation. In this case, the presenter starts by stating his job, *I am a medical doctor*, and giving some of his previous employment history, *I worked for several years as a physician in the Department of Oncology*. He then goes on to mention his position now, *Currently, I am doing research at the Cancer Center Karolinska in the group of Professor Arne Ostman in Stockholm*. Please note that, *I am doing research at + place*, is the same as, *I'm working at + place*.

Here is another example of a presenter providing background information.

> I'm a neuroscientist. My field is psychoneuropharmacology. My current research focuses on schizophrenia, Parkinson's disease and addiction. I'm particularly interested in animal models.

In just four short sentences, the presenter has given the audience all the relevant background information that they need to know. In this example, the speaker first introduces his job by saying, *I'm a neuroscientist*. He then goes on to state his field, *My field is psychoneuropharmacology*. He mentions the research he is doing now, *My current research focuses on schizophrenia, Parkinson's disease and addiction*. Then he is more specific and says, *I'm particularly interested in animal models*.

So the sentence pattern looks like this.

I'm a (   ). My field is (   ). My current research focuses on (   ). I'm working on (   ).

Here is another example of a presenter providing background information.

- *I'm a theoretical chemist. My field is theoretical computational chemistry.*
- *I'm working on computer simulations of protein functions.*

The following three sentences are ways of introducing your research.
- *I'm conducting research on + topic.*
- *I'm doing research on + topic.*
- *I'm working on + topic.*

> **BUT NOT**: *I'm researching on + topic.*
>
> The sentence *I'm researching on semiconductors* is NOT correct.
> You CAN say, *I'm doing research on semiconductors* or *I'm research-ing semiconductors*.
>
> Also, please note the following:
> - *I'm doing research at + place.*
>   Example *I'm doing research at the High Energy Physics Lab.*
> - *I'm doing research on + topic.*
>   Example *I'm doing research on vehicle life-cycle assessment.*

The sentence *My major is + field* is NOT correct as a way to describe your research. It is only correct in terms of a student studying at university. For example, *I'm a sophomore. I'm majoring in psychology* or *I majored in physics at university*.

Key Point

● ゲストスピーカーの場合は，最初に自分の職業，肩書き，研究領域などを紹介すると，聴衆は演者の立場や講演内容が理解しやすくなる．

3. I would like to give a brief introduction to our research field and present our ongoing work.

The presenter then moves on to the topic of the presentation. Notice that he uses the phrase, *give a brief introduction to + topic*.

For more examples using the word *give*, see, Quick Guide 2. Starting your presentation – Key Vocabulary: Page 32, No. 2.

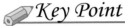

Key Point

- 'give a brief introduction to + topic' を使って，自己紹介から主テーマに移る．

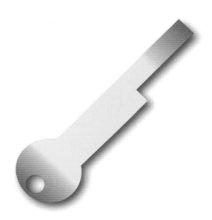

Example introduction 3 (Part 2)

After making some general remarks and introducing himself, the presenter moves on to the first part of his presentation.

Listen to the audio file and read the script.

> Our main subject of interest is best illustrated in this slide. Here you see the histology of four different cancer types. The first picture here shows lung cancer that consists of cancer cells, but there is also a large proportion of non-malignant cells comprising the tumorstroma. This includes inflammatory cells, cells of the vasculature and fibroblasts. These fibroblasts often represent the most abundant cell types in the tumorstroma and are commonly called cancer associated fibroblasts, or in short CAFs. We believe that these CAFs are not only innocent bystanders, but play an important role in cancer development and progression. In the next few slides, I'll show you some experimental evidence for that.

The first thing you will notice is that this example introduction is quite different from example introductions 1 and 2. The speaker does not do any of the following: give a simplified title, an overview of the contents or include any sequence markers, such as first, next, then or in part one. This presentation is different from the above example introductions because it starts with a slide showing the histology of four different cancer cells and not a contents slide. Let's look in detail at what the speaker does and consider how effective it is.

1. Our main subject of interest is best illustrated in this slide.

Using this sentence, the presenter introduces the topic of the presentation with a slide showing the histology of four different types of cancer cells. He does not give a list of contents. The advantage is that the visual image acts as an anchor in the presentation, drawing the audience's attention to the topic.

Key Point

● スライドでイラストを使いながらテーマを紹介すると，イメージによって聴衆の関心をひきつけることができる．

2. Here you see the histology of four different cancer types.

The presenter introduces the slide in a simple and effective way, using the phrase, *Here you see + topic*. The majority of Japanese presenters use the phrase, *This slide shows + topic*. This is correct, but the problem is they overuse it. In terms of frequency, the most common way to introduce a slide is to start with the word here. For example, *Here you see the second stage of the process*. The personal pronouns *you* and *we* are commonly used with *here*, and help to create a more personal effect. In addition to the verb *see*, it is possible to use *have*. For example, *Here we have time plotted against temperature*.

Key Point

● スライドの内容を紹介するときは 'here you see + topic' を使うと効果的である．

3. **These fibroblasts often represent the most abundant cell types in the tumorstroma and are commonly called cancer associated fibroblasts, or in short CAFs. We believe that CAFs are not only innocent bystanders, but play an important role in cancer development and progression.**

The presenter introduces the keyword *fibroblasts*. Notice how he goes on to explain the keyword - *(fibroblasts) are commonly called cancer associated fibroblasts* - and introduces the abbreviation - *in short CAFs* -. He then goes on to state the main point of the presentation like this, *We believe that CAFs are not only innocent bystanders, but play an important role in cancer development and progression.*

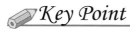 *Key Point*

●キーワードを紹介するときは 'commonly called + topic' を使うとよい.

4. **In the next few slides, I'll show you some experimental evidence for that.**

The presenter introduces the topic for the next few slides. He does it like this. First, he says, *in the next few slides*. He then uses the phrase, *I'll show you some experimental evidence for that*. In other words, before actually showing the slides, he informs the audience of what they are about to see. This is important because it prepares the audience for the information they are about to see.

Here are some examples that can be used to introduce a number of slides connected by a single theme.

- *I'll give you some data about that in the next few slides.*
- *In the next two or three slides, I'll describe our recent experiments.*
- *In the next couple of slides, I'll focus on product development.*

For more information on how to present slides, please see, How to introduce graphics in a dynamic way, on page 64.

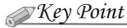 *Key Point*

●スライドを見せる前に何についてのスライドかを知らせるとよい.

In example introductions 1 and 2, we saw how presenters started with a contents slide as part of their introduction. In example introduction 3, we have seen how the presenter started his presentation with an example that acts as an anchor and firmly focuses the attention of the audience on the subject of the presentation. I call this the anchor model. Both methods, the contents slide method and the anchor model, are equally effective. The anchor model is more suitable for presenters who are confident in their English. It does, of course, have one problem: it does not provide an extensive framework of the type provided by a contents slide, as shown in example introductions 1 and 2.

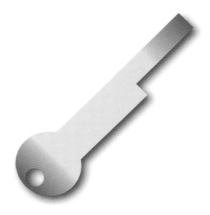

6 Example introduction 4

Some presenters will feel they do not have the time or confidence to follow the example introductions presented above. For those people, I have made a much simpler example introduction that is shorter and easier to use, but equally effective. It only takes about 40 seconds. Here it is. I hope you find it useful. First do listening exercises 1~3. Then read the key sentences.

Listening 1

Listen and match 1~7 with a~g.

1. Today, I'm going to talk about
2. This slide shows
3. As you can see,
4. First,
5. Second,
6. Third,
7. Finally,

a. I'll finish with a brief conclusion.
b. there are four parts
c. a new measuring device.
d. I'll describe some recent results.
e. I'll focus on applications.
f. I'll give a short introduction.
g. the contents of my presentation.

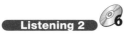

Listening 2

Listen and complete the sentences.

> Today, I'm going to _____ _____a new measuring device. This slide
> _____ the contents of my presentation. As you can see, _____ ____
> four parts. First, I'll _____ a short introduction. Second, I'll _____
> some recent results. Third, I'll _____ _____ applications. Finally,
> I'll _____ _____ a brief conclusion. I'd like to _____ _____
> part one, the introduction.

Listening 3

Listen again. Look at the script and check your answers.

> Today, I'm going to talk about a new measuring device. This slide shows
> the contents of my presentation. As you can see, there are four parts.
> First, I'll give a short introduction. Second, I'll describe some recent re-
> sults. Third, I'll focus on applications. Finally, I'll finish with a brief con-
> clusion. I'd like to start with part one, the introduction.

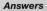

Answers

Listening 1   1-c, 2-g, 3-b, 4-f, 5-d, 6-e, 7-a

Listening 2   talk about, shows, there are, give, describe, focus on, finish with, start
with

27

Example introduction 4
Key Sentences

1. **Today, I'm going to talk about** + (topic).
   Start like this by introducing the topic simply.

2. **This slide shows the contents of my presentation. As you can see, there are four parts.**
   Introduce the contents slide.

3. **First, I'll give** a short introduction.
   Introduce the first topic/part.

4. **Second, I'll describe** some recent results.
   Introduce the second topic/part.

5. **Third, I'll focus on** applications.
   Introduce the third topic/part.

6. **Finally, I'll finish with** a brief conclusion.
   Introduce the last part.

7. **I'd like to start with** part one, the Introduction.
   Move on to part one.

Even if your presentation is only 8 to 10 minutes long, it is possible to include this type of introduction and improve the impact of your presentation considerably. Please remember the point made in the discussion on page 2. *I think you need a framework that shows where you will go in your presentation.* Using the above example, you can easily provide a useful framework for your audience without taking up a lot of time.

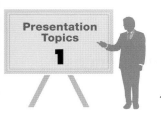

What makes a good presentation?

Every year, we see many presentations, most of which fall into one of three categories. There are some poor presentations, a large number of average presentations and just a few outstanding presentations. But what is it about really excellent presentations that makes them stand out? What do these presentations have that others do not?

One of the ways in which people judge a presentation is by its *degree of novelty*. Presentations that consist mostly of known information are not memorable, whereas the audience will take notice of and remember presentations with a high degree of novelty.

The second point that affects how we view presentations is whether or not we consider them to be *good science*. The term good science refers to the *accuracy of the research and the results* presented. Are we convinced that the approach, methods and experiments are reliable? If there are any flaws in these parts of the research, accuracy will suffer and it cannot be considered to be good science. So *novelty must always be backed up by good science*.

The third point connected with the quality of the presentation concerns *the logic of the presentation and its structure* - by that I mean the *organization of the presentation* and *the way the presenter signals that organization*. For the audience to follow the presentation, it needs to be *accessible and audience-friendly*.

So to summarize, a good presentation should have *novelty, good science,* and *a structure that is accessible and audience-friendly*.

Starting your presentation – Key Sentences

This is a summary of the main points made in this part, along with a list of all the key sentences and vocabulary. It is designed so that you can easily access the information you want and use it to improve your presentation.

❶ *Thanking*

Use these sentences in regular presentations.
- **Thank you, Chairperson.**
- **Thank you very much for your kind introduction.**

Use these sentences in formal situations, such as when you are an invited speaker.
- **It's a great honor to be able to speak to you today.**
- **It gives me great pleasure to speak here today.**
- **I'm very pleased to have the opportunity to present my research at this conference.**
- **I'm delighted to have this chance to present my work here today.**

❷ *Introduce the title / topic of your presentation*
- **Today, I'd like to talk about + topic.**
- **This morning, I want to talk about + topic.**
- **This afternoon, I'm going to talk about + topic.**
- **Today, I'm going to be talking about + topic.**
- **My topic / theme / subject today is + topic.**
- **My presentation today is on / about + topic.**
- **The subject of this presentation is + topic.**

Here are some concrete examples of how to introduce a difficult and complicated title in a simple way. Please remember that your title is already in the conference handbook, the Chairperson will have read it out and it will also appear on your first slide. This means you do not need to read the title again. Instead, you should aim at something much more dynamic, as in the following examples.

Title: Protein tyrosine phosphatases, red-ox-regulated antagonists of receptor tyrosine kinases
Opening: This evening, I would like to talk about the involvement of protein tyrosine phosphatases - an enzyme family - in cell signalling.
Title: Improved Secretion Level of Human Fas Ligand Extracellular Domain by N-terminal Part Truncation in Pichia pastoris
Opening: Today, I'd like to talk about some improvements in the expression and purification of Human Fas Ligand Extracellular Domain.

❸ *Introduce the contents slide / start an overview of your talk*

- This slide shows an outline of my talk.
- As you can see, this slide shows the structure of my presentation.
- This slide shows the contents / structure of my presentation.
- I'd like to start with an overview of my presentation.

❹ *State the number of sections in your talk*

- I'm going to divide my presentation into four parts.
- My presentation is divided into four parts.
- My presentation consists of five parts.
- This presentation is in five parts.
- As you can see, there are four parts in my presentation.

❺ *Using sequence markers to introduce an overview*

- First, second, third, fourth,
- Firstly, secondly, thirdly, fourthly,
- In section one, in section two, in section three, in section four,
- In the first part / section, in the second part / section, in the third part / section, in the last part / section,
- First, then, after that, finally / lastly,

❻ *How to introduce the contents slide / an overview using verbs and just two sequence markers*

It is possible to introduce the contents slide or an overview quite effectively using verbs and just a few sequence markers.

Here is an example using the following verbs: **start with**, **go on to**, **focus on**, **finish with**.

> My presentation is in four parts. I'd like to start with a brief introduction. Then, I'll go on to diagnosis of the disease. After that, I'll focus on possible treatments. I'll finish with a summary of my talk.

Starting your presentation – Key Vocabulary

The following is a list of verbs commonly used in introductions. For each verb introduced, there are several example sentences.

❶ *Talk about*

Talk about is used mainly to introduce the topic of the presentation.
- **Today, I'd like to talk about + topic.**

It is also sometimes used in the middle of the introduction to refer to a topic.
- **In part three, I'd like to talk about possible applications for our new system.**

You cannot say, I'd like to talk about an introduction.

Please do not use the verb talk about more than twice in the introduction to your presentation. It is better to use a variety of different verbs.

❷ *Give*

The verb **give** combines with other words to form a unit.
Here are some common examples.
- **First, I'd like to give a brief introduction to semiconductors.**
- **First, I'd like to give some background information on photosynthesis.**
- **First, I'd like to give a summary of recent developments in the field.**
- **First, I'd like to give you an idea of our latest products.**
- **First, I'd like to give you some results / data from our recent experiments.**
- **First, I'd like to give a review of our recent findings.**
- **First, I'd like to give an outline of how our system can be used in industry.**
- **First, I'd like to give an overview of current methods of treating depression.**

❸ *Introduce*

Here are some examples using the verb **introduce**.
- **In part one, I'd like to introduce two new drugs that can be used in the fight against Parkinson's disease.**
- **After that, I want to introduce several methods of calculating particle size.**
- **Then, I'm going to introduce several new ways of improving efficiency.**

❹ Explain

- Then, I'm going to explain how we collected data.
- In the third part, I want to explain the differences between the old method and the new one.
- I'd like to explain the history of our project and its future development.
- In the last section, I want to explain some of the advantages of the system.

❺ Go on to

- In part three, I'll go on to discuss possible applications.
- After that, I'd like to go on to results and discussion.
- Then, I'll go on to diagnosis of the disease.

❻ Say something about

- In part three, I'd like to say something about our future research plans.
- Next, I want to say something about possible applications.
- Finally, I'm going to say something about how the disease is treated.

❼ Review

- I want to review the major studies in this area.
- I'd like to review some of our recent results.
- I'm going to review the major changes in the field over the last 20 years.
- This is a short review of recent developments in this field.
  (In this sentence, review is used as a noun.)

❽ Look at

- In part two, I'm going to look at modifications to the system.
- Then, I'm going to look at diagnosis and treatment of the disease.
- I'd like to look at two methods of bleaching and compare the results.

❾ *Consider*
- In part three, I want to consider alternatives to current treatments.
- After that, I want to consider several solutions to the problem of side effects.
- I'm going to consider the best way to promote recycling projects in the community.

❿ *Discuss*
- In part two, I'm going to discuss two possible simulations.
- After that, I'd like to discuss the advantages of the new system.
- Finally, I'm going to discuss standard treatment of the disease.

⓫ *Turn to*
- Next, I'll turn to applications of the proposed system in industry.
- After that, I would like to turn to an analysis of our recent results.
- Then, I'm going to turn to the symptoms of the disease and possible treatments.

⓬ *Focus on / Concentrate on*
- I'm going to focus on / concentrate on measurement techniques.
- In part two, I want to focus on / concentrate on two new products.
- Finally, I'd like to focus on / concentrate on possible side effects.

⓭ *Describe*
- In part two, I'm going to describe our latest system.
- Next, I'd like to describe the advantages of the new system.
- I'm going to describe standard treatment of the disease.

⓮ *Mention*
The verb **mention** is generally used to introduce a topic you will talk about briefly.
- In the last part of my presentation, I'd like to mention one or two examples of the system in use in the field.
- After that, I'll mention some of the advantages of the system.
- Finally, I'd just briefly like to mention how we changed the system.

⓯ *Touch on*

The verb **touch on** is generally used to introduce a topic you will talk about briefly.

- **If I have time, I'll touch on some possible applications of the new system.**
- **I'd like to touch on a couple of possible solutions to the problem.**
- **In the last section, I'll touch on diagnosis and treatment.**

⓰ *Finish with*

The verb **finish with** is used to signal the end of your introduction.

- **Lastly, I'll finish with some comments about our future work.**
- **I'll finish with a conclusion.**
- **I'll finish with some remarks about our future research plans.**

⓱ *Summarize*

- **In the last section of this talk, I'll summarize the main findings.**
- **In part five, I'd like to summarize my talk.**
- **Finally, I'll summarize my presentation.**

⓲ *Conclude / Conclusion*

- **I'll conclude my talk with a brief summary of the main points.**
- **In the final part, I'd like to conclude my presentation.**
- **Then, I'll conclude my presentation.**
- **I'll finish with a brief conclusion.**

Presentation Techniques

This discussion is divided into ten short listening exercises. Listen to each part of the discussion, answer the questions and then check the script below. The questions from the discussion are in italics. I hope you enjoy listening to it and find it useful.

※ p. 37 〜 43 **Listening 1 〜 10** の **Answers** は p. 47 に掲載.

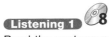

Listening 1

Read the sentences 1~5 below and circle the three points that the speaker makes.

> **Q:** *I'm interested in what makes a good presentation. Can you suggest some of the factors that would influence success?*
>
> For a presentation to be successful, **the presenter must**
> 1. speak loudly and clearly.
> 2. make contact with the audience.
> 3. present material that is understandable and attractive.
> 4. have an attractive handout.
> 5. simplify the material presented.

L: I'm interested in what makes a good presentation. Can you suggest some of the factors that would influence success?

C: Well, it's a very good question. The first point I think is that the presenter should be able to make contact with the audience. That is an essential point. If there is no contact, this will affect the content. The second point is that the presenter has to simplify the material presented. In fact, I think oversimplification is not a problem, as long as this is made clear. The third point is that visualization of the material presented should be understandable and attractive.

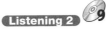

Listening 2

Match the phrases 1~5 with those in a~e.

> **Q:** *Could I just go back to your first point? You said contact with your audience is important. Do you have any specific examples of how you might do that?*
>
> 1. It is important to _____
> 2. The most important thing is _____
> 3. When you point to the screen, _____
> 4. When you look at the audience, _____
> 5. One bit of advice is to _____
>
> a. you should look to the right, left and at the back.
> b. you should turn sideways.
> c. look over the heads of the audience.
> d. never to turn your back on the audience.
> e. look at different people in the audience.

L: Could I just go back to your first point? You said contact with your audience is important. Do you have any specific examples of how you might do that?

C: First of all, it is important to look at different people in the audience. The most important thing is never to turn your back on the audience. When you point to the screen, you should turn sideways. Also, when you look at the audience, you should look to the right, left and at the back. One bit of advice is to look over the heads of the audience.

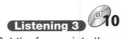

Put the four points the speaker makes in the correct order a~d.

> **Q:** *Okay, let me move on to my second question. I think you have seen a lot of presentations given by Japanese scientists. What are your general impressions of those presentations?*
>
> 1. They do not make a hierarchy of points that are most relevant and less relevant. _____
> 2. Many of them seem to lack confidence. _____
> 3. They present everything as relevant. _____
> 4. They are unable to give an overview of the topic. _____

L: Okay, let me move on to my second question. I think you have seen a lot of presentations given by Japanese scientists. What are your general impressions of those presentations?
C: First of all, many of them seem to lack confidence. The second point is that in the vast majority of cases, they are unable to give an overview of the topic.
L: So you are talking about the ability to overview and summarize.
C: Right. Another thing is that they present everything as relevant. In other words, they do not make a hierarchy of points that are most relevant and less relevant.

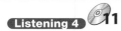**Listening 4**

Circle the four points the speaker makes.

> **Q:** *Some people tell me that they are troubled by Japanese pronunciation. I know you have visited Japan many times. How troubled are you by Japanese pronunciation? How much of a barrier do you think it is in a presentation?*
>
> **Some Japanese presenters**
> 1. make too many grammatical errors.
> 2. do not speak loudly enough.
> 3. have problems with 'l' and 'r'.
> 4. speak too quickly.
> 5. do not project their voice.
> 6. do not pronounce chemical compounds correctly.
> 7. do not stress words or important points.
> 8. speak very well in regular conversation, but seem to have problems in presentations.

L: Some people tell me that they are troubled by Japanese pronunciation. I know that you have visited Japan many times. How troubled are you by Japanese pronunciation? How much of a barrier do you think it is in a presentation?
C: Well, of course, it varies. Some people do not speak loudly enough. Second, they do not project their voice, and they do not stress words or important points. Perhaps this is due to lack of confidence. Some people speak very well in regular conversations, but seem to have problems in presentations.

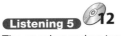

Listening 5 🎧12

The speaker makes ten points about introductions. Listen and put them in the correct order a~j. Letters a,e and j are done for you.

Q: *Okay. I'd like to move on to the next question. I'm thinking of the various parts of a presentation, particularly the introduction. Is an introduction necessary?*

1. Sometimes your presentation will be made up of five distinct parts. _____

2. And at the end, you repeat all the conclusions of each distinct set of data. ___j___

3. An introduction is absolutely necessary. ___a___

4. Then, you go on to explain the methods. _____

5. And you end up with the conclusion. _____

6. What you do is to explain the structure of your presentation and the points to be discussed. _____

7. So you get methods, results, discussion and conclusion five times over. _____

8. After the introduction, you need to introduce the topic and attract the attention of the audience. _____

9. Then, the data. And then, the discussion. ___e___

10. If you have five distinct sets of data, you have to repeat the above. _____

L: Okay. I'd like to move on to the next question. I'm thinking of the various parts of a presentation, particularly the introduction. Is an introduction necessary?

C: Oh, yes. An introduction is absolutely necessary. What you do is to explain the structure of your presentation and the points to be discussed. That is very important. But after the introduction, you need to introduce the topic and attract the attention of the audience. Then, you go on to explain the methods. Then, the data. And then, the discussion. And you end up with the conclusion. Sometimes your presentation will be made up of five distinct parts. If you have five distinct sets of data, you have to repeat the above. So you get methods, results, discussion and conclusions five times over. And at the end, you repeat all the conclusions of each distinct set of data.

L: So you have five mini-conclusions and come up to a major conclusion at the end.

C: Right.

L: That's interesting. What would you say to a presentation that does not have sections?

C: It's like the surface of the ocean. Flat!

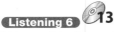 **Listening 6** 13

Listen to this discussion about handling slides. Put the sentences 1~5 in the correct order a~e.

Q: You mentioned in the beginning that presentations should have good slides. Is there any advice for handling slides?

1. And in my case, the next slide is often the conclusion. _____

2. Then, you show the slide. _____

3. Yes, and repetition of the main conclusion is important. _____

4. You have to explain what is on the slide. _____

5. Before the slide appears on the screen, you tell the audience what is on the slide. _____

L: Right! Okay, just a couple of other things. You mentioned in the beginning that presentations should have good slides. Is there any advice for handling slides?

C: Yes, the first thing is that before the slide appears on the screen, you tell the audience what is on the slide. That is very important. Then, you show the slide. And, of course, you have to explain what is on the slide. And in my case, the next slide is often the conclusion.

L: So, you have three steps or stages.

C: Yes, and repetition of the main conclusion is important.

L: Yes, I've seen you use that technique in your presentations and it makes it very user-friendly.

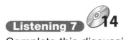

Complete this discussion about effective conclusions by choosing appropriate phrases from 1~7. The first one, a, is done for you.

Q: Okay. Let's move on to conclusions. You said you might have five mini-conclusions and a final conclusion. Do you have any advice for giving good conclusions?

C: Not for the conclusions, per se, but, if possible, you should also explain ____a____ the ____b____. So, let's give an example. I can do research on the snail, and this, of course, is an extremely small piece in the whole field of science, but if I am able to____c____ to other species, that is ____d____ that underlies the importance for people ____e____.

L: So, this is the application of your research. Okay, if I can be a bit more specific, in a conclusion slide or final slide, how many main points would you have?

C: The advice is____f____. The best ____g____!

1. would be one   _____
2. impact of your data   _____
3. outside the snail research community   _____
4. as few as possible   _____
5. generalize some of my findings   _____
6. the impact   _____
7. after the conclusion   ____a____

L: Okay. Let's move on to conclusions. You said you might have five mini-conclusions and a final conclusion. Do you have any advice for giving good conclusions?

C: Not for the conclusions, per se, but, if possible, you should also explain after the conclusion the impact of your data. So, let's give an example. I can do research on the snail, and this, of course, is an extremely small piece in the whole field of science, but if I am able to generalize some of my findings to other species, that is the impact that underlies the importance for people outside the snail research community.

L: So, this is the application of your research. Okay, if I can be a bit more specific, in a conclusion slide or final slide, how many main points would you have?

C: The advice is as few as possible. The best would be one!

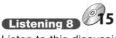

Listen to this discussion about ways of handling questions and surviving the question and answer session. Put these techniques in the correct order a~f. The first one, a, is done for you.

> **Q:** *Okay, that's interesting. I'm just coming up to the last couple of questions. When I'm working with Japanese presenters, trying to help them improve their presentations, the same question comes up every time. How do I handle the Q and A session? How do I survive the Q and A?*
>
> 1. Another important thing is that you must be honest. In other words, you have to say when you don't know the answer. _____
> 2. There are two tricks. The first one is to slowly repeat the questions. This gives you some time to think. ___a___
> 3. You have to know the weak points of your own presentation. So, you prepare all the answers for the weak points. _____
> 4. In case you don't know the answer, you should slightly reshape the question. _____
> 5. One bit of advice is to prepare answers to questions beforehand and make slides. I always have a few slides that I can show after the final slide. _____
> 6. Another thing is to have phrases like: That's a very good question or I'm glad you asked that. _____

L: Okay, that's interesting. I'm just coming up to the last couple of questions. When I'm working with Japanese presenters, trying to help them improve their presentations, the same question comes up every time. How do I handle the Q and A session? How do I survive the Q and A?

C: There are two tricks. The first one is to slowly repeat the questions. This gives you some time to think. That's good when you know the answer. In case you don't know the answer, you should slightly reshape the question.

L: Yes, I saw you do that in your last presentation.

C: Yes, that's what I tell my PhD students to do. Another thing is to have phrases like: That's a very good question or I'm glad you asked that.

L: I see a lot of Japanese presenters who cannot use those kinds of techniques and they freeze.

C: Yes, they get stuck. One bit of advice is to prepare answers to questions beforehand and make slides. Maybe you have noticed, I always have a few slides that I can show after the final slide. So in case someone wants to know some more information, you can easily present that slide.

L: So you predict questions.

C: Yes.

L: How do you do that?

C: First of all, you have to know the weak points of your own presentation. So, you prepare all the answers for the weak points. As I have said, you can reshape questions a little and avoid trouble in that way. Another important thing is that you must be honest. In other words, you have to say when you don't know the answer. Or you can say, this is a problem we have been thinking about for a long time, but we haven't found an answer.

L: Is that acceptable?

C: Yes, perfectly acceptable. There's no problem.

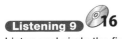

Listening 9 🔘16

Listen and circle the five points the speaker made.

Q: *Another question is how to survive the banquet. What do scientists talk about at the banquet?*

1. Where are you from?
2. Everything, except science. In general, you don't discuss science.
3. Did you see any good presentations?
4. How long did it take to get here?
5. What did you think of the plenary?
6. How was your trip?
7. What are your interests?
8. What is the focus of your research?

L: Another question is how to survive the banquet. What do scientists talk about at the banquet?
C: Everything, except science. In general, you don't discuss science. You might ask: What are your interests? What is the focus of your research? As for general questions, you might ask: How was your trip? How long did it take to get here?

Listening 10 🔘17

Complete the blanks a~f by choosing the best phrases from 1~6.

Q: *This is absolutely the last question. What advice do you have for young Japanese researchers who really want to improve their presentation techniques?*

C: I think it is important to practice your presentation _____a_____. So, when you have got your presentation together, select a group of coworkers and _____b_____. Have them _____c_____. Then, afterwards, _____d_____, _____e_____ and _____f_____.
L: Thanks very much. It has been very interesting talking to you.

1. try out your presentation   _____
2. ask questions   _____
3. in front of your peers   _____
4. the slides   _____
5. the techniques   _____
6. discuss the content   _____

L: This is absolutely the last question. What advice do you have for young Japanese researchers who really want to improve their presentation techniques?
C: I think it is important to practice your presentation in front of your peers. So, when you have got your presentation together, select a group of coworkers and try out your presentation. Have them ask questions. Then, afterwards, discuss the content, the slides and the techniques.
L: Thank you very much. It has been very interesting talking to you.

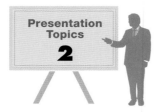

If you could get people to do one thing differently in their presentation, what would it be?

18

I teach several presentation skills classes each week. The participants are all smart people, with promising careers in science who have published papers and presented in English at international conferences. After I have seen their presentations, I always try to give some concrete advice on how to improve for next time. Here, I introduce the things I frequently tell people to do differently. I hope you find them interesting and that you are able to use some of them in your presentations.

1. Have an anchor at the beginning of your presentation

Many presenters provide examples of the application of their research, pictures of sites, machines, technical setups, and so on. But, where do they put these examples? Many people put them at the end of their presentations, almost as if they are some kind of afterthought. This is a mistake. These examples all help to anchor the presentation and give the audience something concrete to visualize and should be at the beginning of your presentation, as part of a brief overview or introduction. Changing the position of these examples from the end to the beginning of the presentation can have a huge impact. For an example of an anchor used effectively at the beginning of a presentation, see example introduction 3 (part 2) on pages 22~25.

2. You are here!

In the street outside most train stations in Japan, there are boards with maps of the area showing roads and buildings. Have you ever used one? What did you look for first? It's almost certain that the first thing you looked for is the little sign, mostly in red, saying 'You are here'. Without that information, you have no idea where you are and have no way of getting to your destination. In a sense, watching a presentation is much like exiting a train station in a place you are not familiar with. You need a map to know where you are. This means that as a presenter, you should remember to signal your location in your presentation. You can do this by providing a good overview as part of your introduction and by indicating movement within the presentation. I have already said how important it is to have a framework in your presentation. A framework acts like a map and guides the audience through your presentation. During your presentation, it is important to signal where you are now and also where you are going.

3. Good visuals are only half the battle: you also need to be able to explain what is in your slides

Slides are a visual media and that means people access information by looking at something. With POWERPOINT©, it is possible to present your data visually in a way that the audience can follow easily. Presenters put a lot of effort into producing high quality slides and in my experience are generally successful. But in addition to creating high quality slides, you need to be able to explain what is in the slide: this is the verbal or spoken element of the slide which is equally important as the visual element. Without adequate explanation your audience will find it difficult to process the data you are presenting. So don't forget to spend time preparing what you are going to say and how you are going to say it, because it's as important as making a great slide.

4. Try to use questions in your presentation

I constantly try to get people to improve their presentations by using questions. This is a simple technique that is commonly used by native speakers to focus on important information and bring a change of pace in the presentation. Japanese presenters rarely use questions in their presentations. In some presentations I see, there are points where a question could easily be used. For example, I recently saw a young researcher talking about the advantages and disadvantages of a new system. He introduced a slide containing a list of the advantages and disadvantages and simply read through each of them. He could have started his slide by saying: *What are the advantages of this system?* When he had finished talking about the advantages, he could have introduced the disadvantages simply and dynamically by saying: *How about the disadvantages?* It's simple and effective. Why not try and include at least a couple of questions in your next presentation? I think you'll find it really makes a difference.

5. Grammar advice: Use active and not passive sentences

The following two sentences have different grammar patterns, but the same meaning.

The sample was heated to 25 degrees.
We heated the sample to 25 degrees.

The first of the two sentences above is in the passive voice and is more appropriate for a scientific paper or a laboratory report. For an oral presentation, it is too formal and overloads the audience. It is much easier and more effective to use an active sentence and say, *We heated the sample to 25 degrees.* The problem is, however, that non-native speakers tend to use passive sentences in oral presentations a lot more than native speakers. Recent research has shown that non-native speakers use the passive 30 percent more than native speakers.

Another advantage of using active sentences is that you can use the personal pronouns 'I', 'you' or 'we' which creates a sense of joint effort and belonging in the audience. Use of the passive, however, creates an impersonal effect closer to the research article than the oral presentation, and results in a less interactive presentation. So, my advice to you is to avoid passive sentences in your presentations. Instead, use active sentences which create an informal, lighter atmosphere that includes the audience.

6. It is important to have some movement within your presentation

Another difference between presentations given by native and non-native speakers is in the amount of movement within the presentation. Non-native speakers tend to move in a straight line from introduction through to conclusion; this is probably because of the pressures of speaking in a foreign language. Native speakers, however, tend to use forward and backward movement in their presentations to help guide the audience.
Typical sentences for forward movement are:

I'll talk about that later.
I'll show you that information in the next slide.

And for backward movement, typical sentences are:

I'd like to go back to the data in slide 2.
I'd like to remind you of the data I showed you in the first few slides.

7. Slow down! It is not a race

Most presenters tend to rush through their presentations. They do not give their audience the time to take in the information they are presenting. This is particularly true of the conclusion section. I see a lot of presentations where people rush through the conclusion and consequently create a poor impression. It is important to pause after each point that you make in the conclusion. A pause of only a few seconds can make a huge difference.

8. Your conclusion is as important as your introduction

Some people rush the conclusion, or simply show a conclusion slide with several points and say nothing. Both of these are poor ways of finishing a presentation and create a very flat ending. When preparing your presentation, one piece of advice is to spend as much time preparing the conclusion as you do the introduction. Very often the conclusion slide looks as if the presenter ran out of time. I often say the following things to presenters. You should have put more effort into the conclusion. You should not have rushed. You should not have written in full sentences, but instead have used notes. What I mean is that the presenter needed to spend more time preparing the conclusion.

Answers (p. 37~43)

Listening 1	2, 3, 5
Listening 2	1-e, 2-d, 3-b, 4-a, 5-c
Listening 3	1-d, 2-a, 3-c, 4-b
Listening 4	2, 5, 7, 8
Listening 5	1-g, 2-j, 3-a, 4-d, 5-f, 6-b, 7-i, 8-c, 9-e, 10-h
Listening 6	1-d, 2-b, 3-e, 4-c, 5-a
Listening 7	1-g, 2-b, 3-e, 4-f, 5-c, 6-d, 7-a
Listening 8	1-f, 2-a, 3-e, 4-b, 5-d, 6-c
Listening 9	2, 4, 6, 7, 8
Listening 10	1-b, 2-c, 3-a, 4-e, 5-f, 6-d

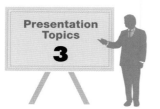

No two specialists are alike

19

Most books on presentation skills give the following advice: *know your audience*. This is reasonable advice, but it is actually difficult to put into practice. If, for example, you are giving a presentation at an academic meeting, I think it is safe to assume that people in the audience will have levels of knowledge similar to your own. But you can never be sure about this, and perhaps *the biggest danger is to assume too much*.

In fact, it is very easy to assume too much about your audience. For example, we imagine that everyone is familiar with the material we are presenting and, therefore, there is no need for an introduction or an overview. We might also skip definitions of technical terms and decide not to simplify difficult information or summarize the main points at the end of sections. We do this because we think everyone knows this information. We also do it because we want to save time and introduce more important data.

This is a mistake. *In every presentation, you need some kind of an introduction or overview that acts as a map for the audience. You also need to define technical terms, simplify difficult information, and summarize the main points at the end of sections*. The reason for this is that even in a fairly homogenous audience at an international conference, *no two specialists will be alike*. This is because each one of the people in the audience approaches the subject from a slightly different angle and, accordingly, has a different focus. So, when we prepare our presentations, it is worth keeping in mind that *no two specialists are alike*.

Part 2

How to handle the main body of your presentation

In this part, I want to make some suggestions that will help you to improve the connectivity of the main body of your presentation. What do I mean by connectivity? I'm referring here to the way in which the presenter signals the structure of the presentation, and also how the information presented is linked.

I'm also going to consider transparency. By transparency, I mean ways of making your presentation as clear as possible for the audience by using appropriate English to stress important points and focus on key data.

Here I will introduce some useful sentences to help you improve both the connectivity and transparency of your presentation.

1 Starting a new section

I n the presentations I see, a lot of presenters fail to tell the audience when they are moving on to a new section.

Here are some examples of how to start a new section. The keywords are underlined. Using these sentences will significantly improve the connectivity of your presentation.

- *Now, I would like to move on to the results and discussion section.*
- *Next, I want to go on to part three of my presentation and focus on computer simulations.*
- *Let's take a look at some of the data from the second series of experiments we conducted.*
- *I would now like to turn to part two of this presentation and consider the advantages of the new system I have introduced.*
- *Okay, so I've mentioned all the symptoms of the disease. Now, I am going to have a look at possible treatments for depression.*

Please note that the while the expressions *take a look at* and *have a look at* are widely used in oral presentations they are too informal for written scientific papers and are generally not used.

Also, note that *move on to* and *go on to* have exactly the same usage. The verbs *take a look at* and *have a look at* also have the same usage.

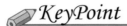 *KeyPoint*

●新しいセクションに移るときは，上記のフレーズを用いると講演内容に流れができて質が上がる．

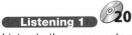

Listening 1 20

Listen to these presenters introducing a new section or part of their presentation. Which verbs do they use? Put the verbs in the correct order a~e.

1. move on to _____
2. go on to _____
3. take a look at _____
4. turn to _____
5. have a look at _____

Listening 2 20

Now listen again and complete the sentences.

a. Next, I would like to _____ _____ part three of my presentation.
b. Now, I'd like to _____ _____ _____ _____ the experimental setup.
c. Now, I'm going to _____ _____ _____ the results and discussion part of my presentation.
d. Okay, let's _____ _____ _____ _____ data from the second series of experiments.
e. Now, I want to _____ _____ _____ part two.

Script
a. Next, I would like to turn to part three of my presentation.
b. Now, I'd like to take a look at the experimental setup.
c. Now, I'm going to move on to the results and discussion part of my presentation.
d. Okay, let's have a look at data from the second series of experiments.
e. Now, I want to go on to part two.

Answers
Listening 1 1-c, 2-e, 3-b, 4-a, 5-d
Listening 2 a.turn to, b.take a look at, c.move on to, d.have a look at, e.go on to

2 Focusing on important points in a section

Ⅰ n a presentation, we deal with a large amount of data that the audience needs to process in order to follow what we are saying. To help the audience, we need to emphasize the most important information in our presentation. This is sometimes referred to as the take home message. In some cases, this will involve simplifying data so that the main points are understandable. In fact, as pointed out in Presentation Techniques: Discussion on page 37, Listening 1, oversimplification is not a problem, as long as it helps the audience to understand the data that is being presented. If we simplify our data, it will significantly improve the transparency of our presentation.

Think what happens if you do not emphasize or simplify; all the information in your presentation is presented as equally relevant and the main points are not stressed. Consequently, the take home message is weak and your presentation is difficult to understand. The audience is left asking these questions: What did the presenter want to say? What were the main points of the presentation?

When I see Japanese presenters presenting in Japanese, I see very little evidence of emphasis or simplification in their presentations and, consequently, transparency suffers. This means they do not stress the main points and do not create a hierarchy of points or indicate the relative importance of data. When I see the same people presenting in English, I see exactly the same problems. They have good data, great slides and reasonably good English: the problem is they fail to make their presentations audience-friendly because they do not emphasize enough and, consequently, transparency fails.

Here are some examples of how to emphasize important information within a section.

- *I would like to emphasize that although this computer simulation takes much longer, it achieves a greater degree of accuracy.*
- *I want to draw your attention to this set of data which suggests this system has several advantages.*
- *I would like to stress that although we have a lot of data, we are still unsure how the mechanism works.*
- *My main point is that we can improve the performance of this system by making the changes I have mentioned here.*
- *I would like to point out that the rate of increase shown in Figure 1 is twice that of the previous experiment.*

KeyPoint

●重要な情報やデータを示すときは，それを強調したり簡単に説明したりしないと，聴衆は理解しにくい．

Listening 1

Listen to these presenters emphasizing important information within a section. Which phrases do they use? Put them in the correct order a~e.

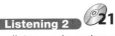

1. to emphasize that   _____
2. to draw your attention to _____
3. to stress that   _____
4. my main point is that   _____
5. to point out that   _____

Listening 2

Now listen again and complete these sentences.

a. I'd like to _____ _____ these are just interim conclusions. Further experiments are necessary.
b. I'd like to _____ _____ _____there is a melting peak at this point.
c. I want to _____ _____ _____ to the trade figures for 2009.
d. I want to _____ _____ this method has three main advantages compared to the previous method.
e. _____ _____ _____ _____ _____ with recent advances in drug development, the outlook for these patients is much better.

Script
a. I'd like to stress that these are just interim conclusions. Further experiments are necessary.
b. I'd like to point out that there is a melting peak at this point.
c. I want to draw your attention to the trade figures for 2009.
d. I want to emphasize that this method has three main advantages compared to the previous method.
e. My main point is that with recent advances in drug development, the outlook for these patients is much better.

Answers
Listening 1 1-d, 2-c, 3-a, 4-e, 5-b
Listening 2 a.stress that, b.point out that, c.draw your attention, d.emphasize that, e.My main point is that

3 Finishing sections with a short summary

In most presentations, summaries of the main points come in the conclusion. However, it is becoming increasingly common to give short summaries at the end of sections, particularly if the information presented is dense and the load on the audience heavy. (See, for example, Presentation Techniques : Discussion on page 39, Listening 5). Of course, you do not need to summarize at the end of every section. However, if you do this some of the time, it will make your presentation more accessible for the audience.

Here are some examples of how to summarize the main points at the end of a section.

- *I'd like to summarize the advantages of the new system I've introduced in this section.*
- *These are the key points. First, ... Second, ... Third, ...*
- *At this point, I'd just like to go over the main points.*
- *This is a brief summary of the main points in this section. First, ... Next, ...*

KeyPoint

●セクションの終わりに簡単なまとめを入れると，わかりやすい講演になる．

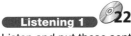

Listening 1 22

Listen and put these sentences in the order that you hear them a~e.

1. Okay, this is just a quick summary of the key points again. _____
2. To finish this section, I'll just mention the main points. _____
3. Okay, these are the main points that I made in section two. _____
4. To summarize, these are the main points that I made in this section.

_____
5. I'll finish this section by going over the main points again. _____

Script
a. I'll finish this section by going over the main points again.
b. Okay, this is just a quick summary of the key points.
c. To summarize, these are the main points that I made in this section.
d. Okay, these are the main points that I made in section two.
e. To finish this section, I'll just mention the main points.

Listening 2 23

Listen to these sentences 1~10. Circle the sentences where the presenter
gives a short summary.

1, 2, 3, 4, 5, 6, 7, 8, 9, 10

Script
1. In the next section, I'd like to focus on improvements to the system.
2. I'll go over the key points again.
3. Today, I'd like to talk about biodegradable polymers.
4. I'd like to finish this section by going over the main points.
5. If I have time, I'll touch on some possible applications of the system.
6. These are the main points.
7. Now, I'd like to move on to the results and discussion section.
8. This is a brief summary of this section.
9. I'd like to stress that this data was collected over a period of 2 weeks.
10. I'll just mention the main points again.

Answers
Listening 1 1-b, 2-e, 3-d, 4-c, 5-a
Listening 2 2, 4, 6, 8, 10

4 Signaling the end of a section

In section 1, I stressed the need to signal when you move on to a new section. It can also be helpful to signal the end of a section, particularly if you do not intend to summarize the main points. Signaling the end of the section will help to improve the connectivity of your presentation.

Here are some examples.

- *That covers the experimental setup.*
- *That concludes this section on data collection.*
- *That's all I have to say about initial treatment.*
- *That's the end of this section.*

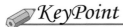 **KeyPoint**

● セクションの終わりに上記のフレーズを用いると講演の質が上がる.

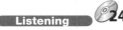 **Listening** 24

Put the sentences 1~4 in the order that you hear them a~d.

1. That covers the experimental setup.	_____
2. That concludes this section on data collection.	_____
3. That's all I have to say about initial treatment.	_____
4. That's the end of this section.	_____

Script
a. That's the end of this section.
b. That concludes this section on data collection.
c. That's all I have to say about initial treatment.
d. That covers the experimental setup.

Answers
1-d, 2-b, 3-c, 4-a

5 Movement within a presentation

A nother way in which the presentation style of native speakers and that of Japanese speakers of English differs is in the movement that takes place within their presentations. With Japanese presenters, I find that the direction is linear, moving from introduction to conclusion in a straight, uninterrupted line, with no forward movement, backward movement, skipping information, or explaining more simply. This puts more pressure on the audience, since they have just one chance to catch the main points. The information is presented at speed and this, too, increases the level of difficulty for the audience.

In this section, I will focus on a number of sentences that you can use for forward movement, backward movement, skipping information and explaining more simply. All of these sentences will help you to improve the movement in your presentation and make it more accessible for the audience.

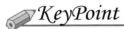
KeyPoint

● 意図的に話題を前後させたり，詳細を省いたり，簡単に言い換えたりすると，講演に動きができる.

Here are some examples.

Forward movement

- *I'll talk about alternative treatments in the next section.*
- *I'll give you more examples of how we collected data in section three.*
- *I'll mention this issue again later.*
- *I'm going to return to that point in section four.*

Backward movement

- *As I already pointed out, samples were measured again at day two of the experiment.*
- *As I already mentioned, we collected data at five different locations in the field.*
- *As I already said, samples were stored at room temperature.*
- *I'd like to refer back to what I said about sample preparation.*

Skipping information

- *Time is limited, so I'll skip that data.*
- *We only have a few minutes left, so I won't go into details.*
- *I won't discuss this in detail.*
- *As time is limited, I'll skip that information.*

Explaining simply

- *In other words, we can increase the yield by several percent with this method.*
- *To put it simply, the rate of increase is approximately twice that of the first experiment.*
- *Basically, the catalytic reaction proceeds at a faster rate than in experiment one.*
- *What I'm saying here is that side effects can be significantly reduced.*

For more information on explaining simply, please see Presentation Topics 9 on page 106.

Listening 1 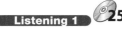 25

You will hear ten sentences. What is the function of each sentence? Write FM for forward movement, BM for backward movement, SI for skipping information and ES for explaining simply.

| 1. _____ | 2. _____ | 3. _____ | 4. _____ | 5. _____ |
| 6. _____ | 7. _____ | 8. _____ | 9. _____ | 10. _____ |

Listening 2 25

Listen again and complete the sentences you hear.

1. I'll _____ _____ more information about that in the next section.
2. _____ _____ _____ _____, we noticed a significant increase in temperature at day two of the experiment.
3. As you can see, there are a large number of equations. So, _____ _____ _____ information.
4. _____ _____ _____, patients in group one seemed to respond more quickly to the drug.
5. I'll _____ _____ that more in the last part of my presentation.
6. As I _____ _____ _____, we found a significant increase at day two of the experiment.
7. I won't _____ _____ _____ on that point.
8. I'll _____ you _____ _____ that later on.
9. This is quite complex. So _____ _____ the details.
10. What _____ _____ _____ is that side effects can be significantly reduced.

Script
1. I'll give you more information about that in the next section.
2. As I already mentioned, we noticed a significant increase in temperature at day two of the experiment.
3. As you can see, there are a large number of equations. So, I'll skip that information.
4. In other words, patients in group one seemed to respond more quickly to the drug.
5. I'll talk about that more in the last part of my presentation.
6. As I already pointed out, we found a significant increase at day two of the experiment.
7. I won't go into details on that point.
8. I'll tell you more about that later on.
9. This is quite complex. So I'll skip the details.
10. What I'm saying here is that side effects can be significantly reduced.

Answers
Listening 1 1-FM, 2-BM, 3-SI, 4-ES, 5-FM, 6-BM, 7-SI, 8-FM, 9-SI, 10-ES
Listening 2 1.give you, 2.As I already mentioned, 3.I'll skip that, 4.In other words, 5.talk about, 6.already pointed out, 7.go into details, 8.tell, more about, 9.I'll skip, 10.I'm saying here

6 Using questions in the main body

I n order to create a dynamic presentation, many presenters, particularly native speakers, use questions. These are called <u>rhetorical questions</u> and are used to focus on important information. Such questions also introduce a change of pace in your presentation and, as such, are extremely useful in the main body of the presentation, as this is the longest section. Questions also improve the transparency of the presentation. However, please note that questions of the type introduced here are <u>not generally used in written scientific papers.</u>

Here are some examples.

- *How can we apply this new method?*
- *What does this result tell us about the mechanism?*
- *How can we interpret this data?*
- *Can the setup be used in other situations?*

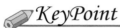
KeyPoint

●疑問形を用いると，講演のリズムを変えることができ，特に長い講演では有益であるし，講演内容のポイントもわかりやすくなる．

Listening 1 — 26

Listen and put these questions in the order that you hear them a~j.

1. How can we solve this problem? _____
2. What are the reasons for this sudden drop in temperature? _____
3. Is it possible to use the system in other situations? _____
4. What about the remaining compounds? _____
5. How far does the new system solve these problems? _____
6. To what extent does the use of the new catalyst improve the reaction?
_____
7. What happens if we adjust the dosage of the drug? _____
8. Are there any advantages in reducing the sample size? _____
9. How does this system work with very thin films? _____
10. What is the depth of the substrate? _____

Script
a. What is the depth of the substrate?
b. How far does the new system solve these problems?
c. To what extent does the use of the new catalyst improve the reaction?
d. What are the reasons for this sudden drop in temperature?
e. Is it possible to use the system in other situations?
f. Are there any advantages in reducing the sample size?
g. How does this system work with very thin films?
h. What about the remaining compounds?
i. What happens if we adjust the dosage of the drug?
j. How can we solve this problem?

Listening 2 — 27

Listen to these extracts from presentations and circle the number of questions the presenter uses.

1. (1, 2, 3, 4)	2. (1, 2, 3, 4)	3. (1, 2, 3, 4)
4. (1, 2, 3, 4)	5. (1, 2, 3, 4)	

Script
1. So in today's presentation, I'll be addressing the following questions. What are the best drugs to use? Are there any side effects? And, how far do our recent results go toward development of new and better drugs? I'll also focus on alternative medicine.
2. So that is the picture for the first of the compounds we looked at. What about compound B? What were the results from our experiments? I'd like to address both of those points now. Okay, so what we found was . . .
3. In the first part, I'd like to say something about Parkinson's disease. What is the disease? How is it caused? And, how do we treat it today? Then, I'll go on to give a brief overview of recent developments in the field.
4. With the data we got, we asked ourselves several questions. What is the importance of dosage? And, how far does dosage affect the outcome? Well, one problem we encountered was . . .
5. As you can see, these are the main conclusions of this study. There are, however, several questions that remain. How can the cost of the production process be reduced? And, what can be done to increase product reliability?

7 Contrasting known information and new information

Presenters need to think about how to make their presentations as transparent as possible. One way of doing this is to present information in the following way. First, present information that the audience knows: in other words, data or concepts that are widely known and generally accepted in the field. If you do this, it helps the audience and gives them an anchor. From that point, the presenter can build on this by presenting new information. In other words, you should move from known information to new information.

Here are some examples of how presenters introduce known information.

- *And it is known that if you block the dopamine, you get an increase in activity in the striatum. (+ new information)*
- *We know that this atypical compound in vitro is indeed an agonist. (+ new information)*
- *What we know is that our population is aging, we also know there will be a bigger need for implants. (+ new information)*
- *We know that when you split a planaria, if you wait, a completely new planaria is formed. (+ new information)*
- *We know this enzyme plays a role, but we don't know if it is indispensable or not. (+ new information)*

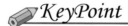*KeyPoint*

●既に知られている情報を先に紹介して，その後に新たな情報を説明する．

Listening 28

Circle the sentences in which the presenter introduces known information.

> 1, 2, 3, 4, 5

Script
1. What does this slide tell us about rates of infection?
2. What we know is that this drug relieves symptoms in over 60 percent of patients.
3. One of the aims of this study was to investigate the effect of aircraft noise on people living near airports.
4. If you look at the table on the right of the slide, you will see an increase in temperature at this point.
5. We know that with this drug, there are some patients who do not respond.

Answers
2, 5

How to introduce graphics in a dynamic way

8

Nowadays, it is easy to produce attractive slides that will help the audience follow your presentation. Having high quality slides, however, does not guarantee success. Presenters have to be able to explain the data contained in their slides. This means that in addition to a strong visual element, the slide itself, the presenter needs a strong oral element, the explanation of the contents of the slide.

On the next page, I am going to introduce three methods of improving the oral element of your slides.

Firstly, I would like to introduce <u>a three-step system for introducing and explaining slides.</u>

Step 1: Introducing the topic / data

Just before the slide comes on the screen, you should tell the audience what they are about to see.

Here are four example sentences.

- *<u>In the next few slides</u>, I'll give you some data on rates of biodegradability.*
- *<u>In the next slide</u>, I'll summarize data from our recent experiments.*
- *I would like to show you some experimental evidence for this <u>in the next couple of slides.</u>*
- *<u>In the next three slides</u>, I'll focus on results from our recent studies.*

Step 2: Explaining the data

When the slide is on the screen, you should introduce the data.

Here are some examples of how to do that.

- *<u>Here we have</u> data from the EU over the last 2 years.*
- *<u>Here you can see</u> a melting peak at this point.*
- *<u>This slide shows</u> rates of cancer in the population.*
- *<u>What we have here is</u> infection rates over the last 10 years in developing countries.*

Step 3: Highlighting important data

You need to focus on important information in the slide.

Here are some examples.

- *<u>I'd like to draw your attention to</u> the sudden increase in values at this point.*
- *<u>I'd like to stress that</u> there are two melting peaks seen here. This is important because . . .*
- *<u>What is interesting here is that</u> values reach a peak at day 20. Then, we see a rapid decline.*
- *<u>The important point here is that</u> values begin to fall at this point.*

This is a summary of the three steps introduced here: <u>first tell the audience what they are going to see, second introduce the data, and third focus on the main points.</u> Of course, you will need to introduce data between these three steps, but with this framework you can be sure that your slides will be easy to follow.

✏️*KeyPoint*

⬤スライドを効果的に活かすためには，①これから見せるものの紹介，②データの説明，③重要な部分の説明，の3ステップで行うとよい．

Method 2

It is important to be able to focus effectively on specific parts of the slide. The most common expression used by Japanese presenters is as follows: _Please look at_ the temperature range. Grammatically, this is correct, but the problem is that some presenters tend to overuse, _'please look at'_. For native speakers, the most common way of focusing on a specific part of the slide is to use the word, _if_.

Here are some examples.

- _If you look at the bar chart on the right, you will see that there is a sudden increase in values at this point._
- _If you look at the data for the second group, you will notice that there are no differences in response._
- _If you look carefully here, you will see a slight improvement in recovery times._
- _If we look on the right side, we see that increased dosage rates do not lead to any improvements._
- _If we look at the right side of this figure, we can see a steep decrease in values._

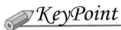 *KeyPoint*

●スライドの重要部分を説明するときは，'if' を使うのも一法である．

Method 3

Finally, I would like to give some examples of how questions can be used as an effective way of explaining your slide. We have already noted on page 60, how the use of questions can help to focus the attention of the audience. They also break up long and detailed explanations. Questions are often used toward the end of the explanation of the slide. The function of the question is to signal the start of a short summary of the main points that were made in the explanation of the data in the slide. They are also useful in focusing the attention of the audience.

Here are some examples.

- _What does this graph tell us about rates of infection?_
- _How can we interpret this data?_
- _What can we conclude from this slide?_

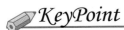 *KeyPoint*

●疑問形を用いることは，スライドの重要部分の説明にも有効である．

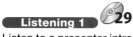

Listen to a presenter introducing and explaining a slide. Which of the following three steps is he using? Circle Step 1 for introducing the topic / data, Step 2 for explaining the data and Step 3 for focusing on important information in the slide.

1. step 1, step 2, step 3
2. step 1, step 2, step 3
3. step 1, step 2, step 3
4. step 1, step 2, step 3
5. step 1, step 2, step 3
6. step 1, step 2, step 3

Script
1.I'd like to draw your attention to the modifications made to the apparatus.
2.Here we have a schematic image of the setup.
3.In the next slide, I'll summarize the main findings of our study.
4.This slide shows the samples at days 2, 5, 7 and 9.
5.In the next four slides, I'm going to introduce data from our recent experiments.
6.What is interesting here is the sudden increase in values at this point.

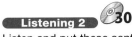

Listen and put these sentences in the order that you hear them a～j. The first one a, is done for you.

1.In the next few slides, I'll introduce details of our recent experiments.

     _____

2.What I'm going to show in the next few slides is various treatments.

     _____

3.This slide shows data on emissions from the EU.   _____

4.Here we have population growth in developing countries.   __a__

5.I'd like to stress that the data in this slide was collected over a period of several years.   _____

6.What is interesting here is that biodegradability rates in samples 1 and 2 are higher than those in samples 3 and 4.   _____

7.If you look at the data shown in the graph on the right, you will see that compound B acts at a faster rate than any other compound.   _____

8.If you look at the right side, you will see a sudden decrease in values.

     _____

9.How can we interpret the data presented here?   _____

10.What does this slide tell us about rates of infection?   _____

Script

a. Here we have population growth in developing countries.

b. I'd like to stress that the data in this slide was collected over a period of several years.

c. What I'm going to show in the next few slides is various treatments.

d. If you look at the right side, you will see a sudden decrease in values.

e. What does this slide tell us about rates of infection?

f. This slide shows data on emissions from the EU.

g. How can we interpret the data presented here?

h. What is interesting here is that biodegradability rates in samples 1 and 2 are higher than those in samples 3 and 4.

i. If you look at the data shown in the graph on the right, you will see that compound B acts at a much faster rate than any other compound.

j. In the next few slides, I'll introduce details of our recent experiments.

Answers

Listening 1   1-step 3, 2-step 2, 3-step 1, 4-step 2, 5-step 1, 6-step 3,

Listening 2   1-j, 2-c, 3-f, 4-a, 5-b, 6-h, 7-i, 8-d, 9-g, 10-e

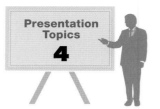

What is obvious to you, may not be obvious to your audience

31

It goes without saying that every presenter knows his or her data thoroughly. This is because each and every day, we do experiments, collect and analyze data, and write lab reports and papers. That is why we know our data so well.

But this presents a problem. We know our data too well, and, consequently, when explaining data in our presentation, we take things for granted. In other words, what is obvious to us is not always obvious to our audience. And this is exactly where our audience gets lost and confused. *So, it is always important to step back and look at our own presentation through the eyes of someone unfamiliar with the material*.

Part 3

How to handle conclusions

In this part, I will focus on how to create effective conclusions. First, I will introduce some general advice with example sentences. Then, I will move on to an analysis of three conclusions from real presentations and introduce some useful techniques and sentences that you can use in your own presentations.

1 Advice for effective conclusions

n this section, I will introduce twelve pieces of general advice for creating effective conclusions.

1. It is important to signal the start of your conclusion clearly.

Use one of these sentences.
- *I'd like to finish by summarizing the main findings of this study.*
- *This is a summary of our results / study / research.*
- *These are the main points of this study.*
- *I want to finish with a short summary.*
- *I'd like to finish / conclude by making the following points.*

The expression, *in conclusion*, is overused. It is a boring way of signaling the start of your conclusion. Try to avoid it and create a more dynamic ending to your presentation by using one of the sentences above.

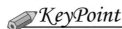

●結論に入るときは，上記のフレーズを用いて結論に移ることを示す．

2. Introduce the main points of your conclusion.

Use one of these sentences.
- *In this study, we found that + main points.*
- *Our results indicate the following. First, … Second, … Third, … Finally, …*
- *This slide summarizes the main findings of this study. Firstly, … Secondly, …Thirdly, … Lastly,…*

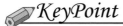

●上記のフレーズを用いて結論のポイントを示す．

3. Do not overload your audience with information in the conclusion.

I once asked a very experienced presenter how many points you should have in a conclusion. He replied, just one. I think he meant this as a joke, but the message was that you should have as little information as possible on the slide, or rather that you should take care not to overload the audience with information in your conclusion. As a general rule, your final slide should not exceed 8 lines.

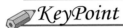

●結論ではあまり多くの情報を詰め込まないようにして，聴衆の負担を減らす．

4. The points on your conclusion slide should be written in note form, not full sentences.

In the following three examples, I will show you how to change a full sentence into note form. I will also show you the English you need to introduce the note form sentence.

Example 1

Full sentence:A new measurement system with increased accuracy was developed.
Note form on slide:New measurement system - increased accuracy
Script:We developed a new measurement system with increased accuracy.

Example 2

Full sentence:It has been shown that a high percentage of waste metals can be recycled.
Note form on slide:High percentage of waste metals → recyclable.
Script:Our study has shown that a high percentage of waste metals can be recycled.

Example 3

Full sentence:It was found that yield increased by over 15 percent.
Note form on slide:Increased yield → over 15 percent
Script: We found that yield increased by over 15 percent.

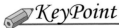

●結論を示すスライドは，フルセンテンスではなく簡単な形式で記載する．

5. Avoid passive sentences in your conclusion.

It is important not to use passive sentences in your conclusion.

This is because the audience can process active sentences more easily than passive ones. Passive sentences are more appropriate for academic papers and lab reports, and are too formal for oral presentations.

Example 1

Passive: Film with a high resolution was obtained.

Active: We got film with a high resolution.

Example 2

Passive: A new automated system was developed.

Active: We developed a new automated system.

Example 3

Passive: It was found that 85 percent of patients responded to the drug.

Active: We found that 85 percent of patients responded to the drug.

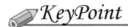 *KeyPoint*

●結論のスライドでは，受動態より能動態を用いるのが好ましい.

6. Do not read the sentences directly from your conclusion slide.

Quite a lot of presenters read each part of their conclusion directly from the slide which creates a boring conclusion. This is a common mistake and is usually caused by using full sentences on the final slide. If you read directly from your conclusion slide, the final part of your presentation becomes flat. The problem lies in the fact that you have complete sentences on your conclusion slide. If you change your complete sentences to notes, as in number 4, this will improve the impact of your conclusion.

KeyPoint

●結論ではただスライドを読み上げることはしない.

7. Simply showing a conclusion slide is not enough.

It is still quite common to see presenters show a conclusion slide and say nothing. They simply wait while the audience reads the points on the slide. This creates a flat ending to the presentation. It is better to have a conclusion in note form and introduce each point using the language introduced in this section.

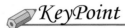 *KeyPoint*

●結論ではただスライドを示すだけでなく，言葉で説明をしたほうがよい．

8. Signal the end of your conclusion clearly.

In number 1 above, I stressed the importance of signaling the start of your conclusion. It is equally important to signal the end of your conclusion clearly. Here are some examples.

* *That's all I have to say. Thank you for your attention.*
* *That concludes my presentation. Thank you.*
* *That covers everything I want to say. Thank you.*
* *Thank you.*

Do not say *that's all* or *finished*. These expressions are not correct in this situation.

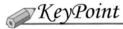 *KeyPoint*

●結論を終えるときは，上記のフレーズを用いてそのことを示す．

For many presenters, this will be end of their presentation. Some presenters, however, will include points 9, 10 and 11. Also, please note that it is possible to use point 8 after points 9, 10 and 11.

9. Refer to your future research plans.

Use one of these sentences.

- *I'd just like to mention our future research plans. We plan to carry out further experiments using different polymers.*
- *The aim of our future work will be to conduct further tests on biodegradability.*
- *The next step in this research is to collate data from the clinical trials and then to think about modifying the system.*
- *The aim of our future work will be to functionally analyze these identified genes and to evaluate them as potential novel targets for anticancer therapy.*

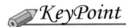KeyPoint

●これからの研究プランに言及するときは上記のフレーズを用いる.

10. Acknowledge your coworkers.

- *In concluding, I would just like to thank my colleagues and collaborators who have contributed to this work. The work on COMT mutants was carried out by several PhD students.* (Show a list of names and / or a photograph).
- *I want to acknowledge our international collaborators in this work. The COMT knockout mice came from the following people at London University.* (Show a list of names and / or a photograph).
- *I would like to acknowledge the people who worked with us on this project.* (Show a list of names and / or a photograph).
- *I want to thank the people who have been involved in this work.* (Show a list of names and / or a photograph).
- *I'd like to mention my coworkers.* (Show a list of names and / or a photograph).
- *Finally, I'd like to acknowledge a lot of people. Most of the work is done by PhD students. This is a list of their names.* (Show a list of names and / or a photograph).

It is common to show a list of names and / or a photograph. Some presenters mention each person individually, others do not.

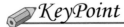KeyPoint

●共同研究者への謝辞は上記のように言う.

11. Acknowledge sources of funding.

Some, but not all, presenters acknowledge sources of funding.

- *We depend a lot on grants. For this project, we are getting funding from the Royal Dutch Academy, the Royal Netherlands Academy of Arts and Sciences, and the Dutch Program for Tissue Engineering.*
- *I'd just like to say that this research was partly funded by the Sato Fund at Nihon University School of Dentistry.*

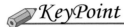**KeyPoint**

● 研究費の提供者への謝辞を言う場合もある.

12. If there is no chairperson present, you should invite questions. Here is how to do it.

- *If you have any questions, I'd be pleased to answer them.*
- *I wonder if anyone has any questions.*
- *I'd like to take questions now.*

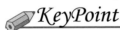**KeyPoint**

● 座長がいないときは, 上記のように質問を受けつける.

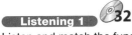
Listen and match the functions 1~7 with the sentences you hear a~g.

1. Signal the start of your conclusion.	_____
2. Introduce the main points of your conclusion.	_____
3. Signal the end of your conclusion.	_____
4. Refer to your future research plans.	_____
5. Acknowledge your coworkers.	_____
6. Acknowledge sources of funding.	_____
7. Invite questions.	_____

Listening 2 32

Listen again and complete these sentences.

a. I'd just like to _____ our _____ _____ _____. We are going to carry out further experiments with different polymers.

b. For this project, we are _____ _____ from the Royal Dutch Academy.

c. I'd like to finish by _____ the _____ _____ of this study.

d. If you have any questions, I'd _____ _____ to answer them.

e. That's all I _____ _____ _____. Thank you for your attention.

f. I _____ _____ _____ the people who have been involved in this work.

g. Our results _____ the following: First, all products tested were effective. Second, there were no reported side effects.

Script

a. I'd just like to mention our future research plans. We are going to carry out further experiments with different polymers.

b. For this project, we are getting funding from the Royal Dutch Academy.

c. I'd like to finish by summarizing the main findings of this study.

d. If you have any questions, I'd be pleased to answer them.

e. That's all I have to say. Thank you for your attention.

f. I want to thank the people who have been involved in this work.

g. Our results indicate the following: First, all products tested were effective. Second, there were no reported side effects.

Answers

Listening 1 1-c, 2-g, 3-e, 4-a, 5-f, 6-b, 7-d

Listening 2 a.mention, future research plans, b.getting funding, c.summarizing, main findings, d.be pleased, e.have to say, f.want to thank, g.indicate

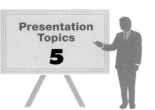

How sticky is your pre-sentation?

33

Some presentations are highly memorable; others we forget quite quickly. What's the difference between a highly memorable presentation and one that is less so? Having great data is certainly one of the keys to creating a presentation that will remain in the minds of the audience, but great data is no guarantee of success. In some cases, even if we present highly novel data, the audience will be thinking: What does this data mean? What is the significance of this data? What point does the presenter want to make? Presenters need to realize that, *even with great data, you have to tell a story that explains the relevance of your data*.

Finally, let's look at the title: How sticky is your presentation? We need to consider the word sticky. If your presentation is sticky, it means it is highly memorable and the audience will be able to recall the data and main points. *Your presentation will only be sticky if you tell a story, connect sections, stress important information and make your data as accessible as possible for your audience*.

2 Example conclusion 1

I am going to introduce three example conclusions. The conclusions presented here can act as models for your own presentations. You can use the key sentences and vocabulary to make your own conclusion more convincing.

Here is a conclusion slide that consists of just three points. It is clear, concise and effective. This is how it appeared, before any changes.

Before revision

> **Conclusion**
> 1. **Technology, which can control cell adhesion by light irradiation, has been developed.**
> 2. **A cell manipulation system, which can make a pattern of cultivated cells at the precision of each cell, has been developed to utilize the above technology.**
> 3. **A prototype of the tailor-made micro-tissue array chip has been developed.**

The points made in the above conclusion are written in full sentences. The sentences are in the passive and the word developed is used three times. With this style, I think there are the following problems.

1. The presenter will probably read the sentences directly from the slide.
2. Full sentences overload the audience.
3. Full sentences reduce the visual impact of the slide.
4. The use of the passive makes the conclusion lack impact.
5. The word developed is repeated too many times.

After revision

> **Conclusion**
> 1. **possible to control cell adhesion by light ir-radiation**
> 2. **possible to make a pattern of cultivated cells using a cell manipulation system**
> 3. **development of a prototype tailor-made mi-cro-tissue array chip**

If we write in note form, the audience can see the main points of our conclusion more easily. But remember that for note form conclusions, the accompanying script is very important. Here is the script for the above note form conclusion.

I'd like to finish my presentation by summarizing the main points. First, using this new technology I presented today, it is now possible to control cell adhesion by light irradiation. (pause) Second, we developed a cell manipulation system. Using this new system, we can make a pattern of cultivated cells. (pause) Third, as I have explained, we developed a prototype tailor-made micro-tissue array chip. (pause) I'd just like to acknowledge my coworkers. This is a list of their names with a photo of our group. Thank you for your attention. (If you have any questions, I'd be pleased to answer them.)

Let's analyze this revised conclusion and consider its good points. The speaker does the following.

Signals the conclusion: I'd like to finish my presentation by summarizing the main points.
Introduces the first point: First, using this new technology I presented today, it is now possible to control cell adhesion by light irradiation.
Introduces the second point: Second, we developed a cell manipulation system. Using this new system, we can make a pattern of cultivated cells.
Introduces the third point: Third, as I have explained, we developed a prototype tailor-made micro-tissue array chip.
Acknowledges coworkers: I'd just like to acknowledge my coworkers. This is a list of their names with a photo of our group.
Thanks the audience: Thank you for your attention.
Invites questions: If you have any questions, I'd be pleased to answer them.

3 Example conclusion 2

N ow let's look at another conclusion. This is how the conclusion slide appeared at first, before any changes.

Before revision

> **Conclusion**
> The results of the studies indicate that dental students using an ergonomically designed seat, such as the Bambach saddle seat have shown reduced muscle work, improved neck posture, decrease of pain, and this may decrease the development of musculoskeletal disorder among dental students.

This conclusion has the following problems.

1. It is difficult for the audience to see the main points of the conclusion easily.
2. It consists of only one full sentence.
3. There are too many redundant words.
4. It is too formal.
5. It has too many lines of text.

All of the above points prevent the audience from understanding the conclusion easily and quickly. This is the revised version. The audience can clearly see three important points followed by the main conclusion.

After revision

> **Conclusion**
> Dental students using an ergonomically designed seat showed
> 1. reduced muscle work
> 2. improved neck posture
> 3. decreased pain
> Use of the seat resulted in a decrease in development of musculoskeletal disorder

Here is the script to accompany the above note form conclusion.

I'd like to finish with a summary of our work. We looked at the effects of using an ergonomically designed seat such as the Bambach saddle seat. Our results showed three main benefits. First, reduced muscle work. Second, improved neck posture. Third, decreased pain. Taking these three benefits together, we found there was a decrease in the development of musculoskeletal disorder in dental students who used the Bambach saddle seat. I'd like to briefly acknowledge the students who participated in this study. I would also like to thank the staff members at the University of Birmingham who assisted in this study. This study was funded by Bambach Saddle Seat Europe Ltd. That's all I have to say. Thank you for your attention. (I'd be happy to answer any questions you might have.)

Let's analyze this revised conclusion and consider its good points. The speaker does the following.

Signals the conclusion: I'd like to finish with a summary of our work.
Reminds the audience of the main aims of the research: We looked at the effects of using an ergonomically designed seat such as the Bambach saddle seat.
Signals the main results: Our results showed three main benefits.
Introduces the results: First, reduced muscle work. Second, improved neck posture. Third, decreased pain.
Introduces the main conclusion: Taking these three benefits together, we found there was a decrease in the development of musculoskeletal disorder in dental students who used the Bambach saddle seat.
Acknowledges coworkers: I'd like to briefly acknowledge the students who participated in this study. I would also like to thank the staff members at the University of Birmingham who assisted in this study.
Acknowledges funding: This study was funded by Bambach Saddle Seat Europe Ltd.
Signals the end of the presentation: That's all I have to say.
Thanks the audience: Thank you for your attention.
Invites questions: I'd be happy to answer any questions you might have.

4 Example conclusion 3

Here is an example of a conclusion that needs no revision. It is clear, concise and the audience can see the main points easily. You can find the introduction to this presentation on page 22.

> **Conclusion**
> 1. Establishment of a reliable method to characterize CAFs
> 2. Identification of CAF specific genes in basal cell cancer
> 3. Observation of similarities and differences to CAFs from other tumor types

Here is the script for the above conclusion.

> I would like to summarize my presentation. Firstly, I showed you that we were able to establish robust and reliable procedures to comprehensively characterize the expression profile of CAFs in individual cancer patients. Secondly, we identified a set of specific genes that were commonly up-regulated in CAFs of basal cell cancer. Finally, we observed similarities, but also differences in the gene signatures of CAFs in different cancer types. The aim of our future work will be to functionally analyse these identified genes and to evaluate them as potential novel targets for anti-cancer therapy. I hope our project will arouse interest in a cell type that has usually not been considered as a main player in tumorigenesis. Thank you very much for your attention.

Let's analyze this conclusion and consider its good points. The speaker does the following.

Signals the start of the conclusion: I would like to summarize my presentation.

Introduces the first point: Firstly, I showed you that we were able to establish robust and reliable procedures to comprehensively characterize the expression profile of CAFs in individual cancer patients.

Introduces the second point: Secondly, we identified a set of specific genes that were commonly upregulated in CAFs of basal cell cancer.

Introduces the final point: Finally, we observed similarities, but also differences in the gene signatures of CAFs in different cancer types.

Refers to future work: The aim of our future work will be to functionally analyze these identified genes and to evaluate them as potential novel targets for anticancer therapy. I hope our project will arouse interest in a cell type that has usually not been considered as a main player in tumorigenesis.

Thanks the audience: Thank you very much for your attention.

Quick Guide 3
How to handle conclusions – Key Sentences

This is a summary of the main points made in this part, along with a list of all the key sentences. It is designed so that you can easily access the information you want and use it to improve your own presentation.

❶ Signal the start of your conclusion
- I'd like to finish by summarizing the main findings of this study.
- This is a summary of our results / study / research.
- These are the main points of this study.
- I want to finish with a short summary.
- I'd like to finish / conclude by making the following points.

❷ Introduce the main points
- In this study, we found that + main points.
- Our results indicate the following. First, … Second, … Third, … Finally, …
- This slide summarizes the main findings of this study. Firstly, … Secondly,…Thirdly, … Finally,…

❸ Signal the end of your conclusion
- That's all I have to say. Thank you for your attention.
- That concludes my presentation. Thank you.
- That covers everything I want to say. Thank you.
- Thank you.

❹ Refer to future research plans
- I'd just like to mention our future research plans. We plan to carry out further experiments using different polymers.
- The aim of our future work will be to conduct further tests on bio-degradability.
- The next step in this research is to collate data from the clinical trials and then to think about modifying the system.
- The aim of our future work will be to functionally analyze these identified genes and to evaluate them as potential novel targets for anticancer therapy.

❺ *Acknowledge coworkers*

- In concluding, I would just like to thank my colleagues and collaborators who have contributed to this work. The work on COMT mutants was carried out by several PhD students. (Show a list of names and / or a photograph).
- I want to acknowledge our international collaborators in this work. The COMT knockout mice came from the following people at London University. (Show a list of names and / or a photograph).
- I would like to acknowledge the people who worked with us on this project. (Show a list of names and / or a photograph).
- I want to thank the people who have been involved in this work. (Show a list of names and / or a photograph).
- I'd like to mention my coworkers. (Show a list of names and / or a photograph).

❻ *Acknowledge sources of funding*

- We also depend a lot on grants. For this project, we are getting funding from the Royal Dutch Academy, the Royal Netherlands Academy of Arts and Sciences, and the Dutch Program for Tissue Engineering.
- I'd just like to say that this research was partly funded by the Sato Fund at Nihon University School of Dentistry.

❼ *Inviting questions*

- If you have any questions, I'd be pleased to answer them.
- I wonder if anyone has any questions.
- I'd like to take questions now.

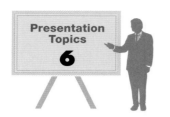

Poster previews

For a long time, poster presentations were considered to be inferior to oral presentations and suitable only for graduate students or young researchers. They were often located in basements or lobbies, sometimes away from the main conference building. But things have changed. *Posters are now an important part of the conference scene and attract a lot more interest than previously.* Some conferences now consist mainly of posters and just a few oral presentations.

One of the advantages of poster presentations is that you can meet face to face with people interested in your poster and discuss the content. Some visitors to your poster will simply be passing through the poster presentation area, others will have seen the summary of your poster in the conference handbook and chosen to visit your poster because it is directly connected with their research.

At a large conference, there can be hundreds of posters and the audience finds it difficult to select the posters they want to see. This is why poster previews have been introduced at some conferences. But what exactly are poster previews? Here is how they work.

Attendees assemble in a large auditorium and watch as each poster presenter gives a mini-oral presentation of 1 or 2 minutes using a single slide or sometimes two. The presenter introduces the content of the poster that he or she will later be presenting. Attendees listen and, depending on the content, decide which posters they will visit.

For presenters, a poster preview is very challenging, since they have to summarize the main points of their research in just one or two slides in the space of a minute or two. This puts pressure on their English skills, as well as their ability to summarize. *This is just another example of how the conference scene is constantly changing, and also of how, as presenters, we continually need to update our skills.*

Part 4

The question and answer session

In this part, I will focus on the question and answer session. It is divided into two sections. 1. How to handle questions and 2. Defining question types.

1 How to handle questions

T he key to a successful question and answer session depends not only on answering questions, but also on controlling the situation and dealing with questions quickly and efficiently. In the first section of this part, I want to introduce twelve key functions for handling questions. I will explain each function and give several examples for each.

1. Asking for repetition

If you didn't catch a question, you can ask for repetition by using one of the following sentences.
- *Excuse me, I didn't catch your question.*
- *Could you repeat that, please?*
- *Would you mind repeating that, please?*

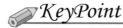KeyPoint

●質問が聞こえなかったときは，上記のように聞きなおす．

2. Asking for clarification

If you didn't understand the meaning or point of a question, you need to ask for clarification.
Here are some useful sentences to use in this situation.
- *Excuse me, I didn't follow your question.*
- *Excuse me, I don't understand your question.*
- *Sorry, I don't follow you.*

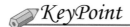KeyPoint

●質問内容がよくわからないときは，わかりやすく言い換えてもらう．

3. Checking the topic

Perhaps you have a general idea of the question, but want to make sure you really understand it before answering. In such a case, you need to check the topic.
- *Is your question about (Figure 3)?*
- *Are you asking about (this data)?*
- *Are you referring to (Figure 2)?*

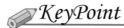KeyPoint

●質問内容に確信がもてないときは，前記のようなフレーズを使って確認する．

4. Checking technical terms

In some cases, the questioner might use a technical term or word you are not familiar with. In this case, you will need to check the meaning of the word.

- *Excuse me, what do you mean by plaque build-up?*

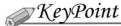 *KeyPoint*

●聞き慣れない専門用語を確認するときは，上記のフレーズを使う．

5. Fielding a question (you want to repeat the question to help the audience)

It is sometimes useful to repeat or summarize the question so that the audience has a chance to hear it again. This technique will help you to keep in control of the question and answer session.

- *Okay, so this is a question about the yield. How much does the yield increase?*
- *We have a question about dosage. What is the best dosage for patients?*

KeyPoint

●質問の内容を繰り返すことで，聴衆も質問内容を再確認でき，演者も頭のなかを整理することができる．

6. Handling unrelated questions

In some cases, people will ask questions that are not directly related to the material you have presented. You can deal politely with unrelated questions by using the following sentences.

- *Unfortunately, that isn't my field. So I can't answer your question.*
- *Sorry, but that is outside the area of this study.*

KeyPoint

●質問の内容が自分の講演内容の対象外のときは，上記のフレーズを使って説明する．

7. Giving a general answer

From time to time, presenters are faced with difficult questions. In such a situation, many presenters tend to hesitate too much and get stuck. One way around this situation is to give a general answer using *basically* or *in general terms*.

- *Basically, we found no significant differences between the two systems.*
- *In general terms, the simulation was successful.*

✐ *KeyPoint*

●難しい質問に対しては，上記のようなフレーズを使って一般論を述べてかわす方法もある．

8. Handling a question you cannot answer

If you are unable to answer a question, it is always better to say so. It is also a good idea to explain why you cannot answer.

- *I'm afraid I can't answer that question. We need more data.*
- *I'm afraid I have no idea, but we are planning to conduct more experiments.*

✐ *KeyPoint*

●答えられない質問を受けたときは，その旨を伝えたり，なぜ答えられないかを説明する．

9. Handling multiple questions (someone asks two or three questions at the same time)

In some cases, people will ask two or three questions at one time. This puts a lot of pressure on you. If you want to remain in control of the situation, you can use these sentences.

- *Okay. I'll take your first question now.*
- *Could I answer your first question now, please?*

✐ *KeyPoint*

●一度に複数の質問を受けた場合は，上記のフレーズを使って1つずつ回答する．

10. Checking the questioner understands / is satisfied with your answer

It is important to check that the questioner understands and is satisfied with your answer. This is called 'checking understanding' and is an essential part of finishing your answer.

- *I hope that answers your question.*
- *Does that answer your question?*
- *Is that okay?*

KeyPoint

●質問に対して答えたときは，上記のフレーズを使って質問者が理解できたかを確認する.

11. Showing you have finished your answer

It is also important to show that you have finished your answer. I am always surprised that so few Japanese presenters do this. You can use the following sentences to signal to the questioner and also the chairperson that you have finished your answer.

- *Thank you.*
- *That's all I have to say on that point.*

KeyPoint

●質問に答え終わったら，上記のフレーズを使ってはっきりとそのことを示す.

12. Asking someone to contact you later

In some cases, it might be possible to get around a difficult situation by inviting the questioner to discuss the problem later. Typically, a presenter would use this technique after first having attempted to answer the question.

- *That is a complicated point. Can we talk about it later?*
- *This is a very complex area. Can we discuss it later?*

KeyPoint

●その場で回答するのが難しいときは，上記のフレーズを使って，あとで直接話す約束をする.

In this section, there are three listening exercises that focus on useful sentences you can use in the Q and A session to help you handle questions easily.

Listening 1   35

First, check that you understand the situations in 1~12 below. Then, listen and match the situations in 1~12 with the sentences you hear a~l. The first one, a, is done for you.

The presenter

1. didn't hear the question _____
2. didn't understand the question _____
3. wants to check the topic of the question _____
4. wants to check a technical term in the question _____
5. wants to repeat the question to help the audience _____
6. deals with a question that is not related to the study _____
7. wants to give a general answer _____
8. cannot answer a question _____
9. wants to stop someone asking several questions at the same time

_____

10. wants to check if the questioner is satisfied with the answer

_____

11. wants to show he / she has finished his / her answer _____
12. asks someone to contact him / her later   a

Script

a. This is a complicated point. I really do not want to go into details. Could we talk about it later?
b. Basically, we found that there is a slight increase in yield.
c. Can I take your first question now, please?
d. I hope that answers your question.
e. I'm afraid we didn't look at that. It wasn't one of the aims of the study.
f. Okay, so this is a question about the catalyst. How fast is the reaction?
g. I'm sorry, I didn't follow your question.
h. I'm sorry, I can't answer that. We do not have enough data.
i. Are you asking about the experimental setup in slide 5?
j. Excuse me, what do you mean by plaque build-up?
k.Thank you.
l. I'm sorry, I didn't catch your question.

Now listen again and complete sentences 1~12.

1. I'm sorry, I didn't _____ your question.
2. I'm sorry, I didn't _____ your question.
3. Are you _____ _____ the experimental setup in slide 5?
4. Excuse me, what do you _____ _____ plaque build-up?
5. Okay, so this is a _____ _____ the catalyst. How fast is the reaction?
6. I'm afraid we didn't _____ _____ that. It wasn't one of the _____ of the study.
7. _____, we found that there is a slight increase in yield.
8. I'm sorry, I can't _____ that. We do not have enough data.
9. Can I _____ your first question _____, please?
10. I _____ that _____ your question.
11. _____ _____.
12. This is a complicated point. I really do not want to go into details. Could we _____ _____ it later?

Script
1. I'm sorry, I didn't catch your question.
2. I'm sorry, I didn't follow your question.
3. Are you asking about the experimental setup in slide 5?
4. Excuse me, what do you mean by plaque build-up?
5. Okay, so this is a question about the catalyst. How fast is the reaction?
6. I'm afraid we didn't look at that. It wasn't one of the aims of the study.
7. Basically, we found that there is a slight increase in yield.
8. I'm sorry, I can't answer that. We do not have enough data.
9. Can I take your first question now, please?
10. I hope that answers your question.
11. Thank you.
12. This is a complicated point. I really do not want to go into details. Could we talk about it later?

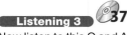
Now listen to this Q and A session. You will hear a member of the audience ask a question and then the reply from the presenter. What is the situation? Match the situations 1~12 with the extracts you hear A~L. The first speaker is the person asking the question and the second speaker the presenter.

> **The presenter**
> 1. didn't hear the question   _____
> 2. didn't understand the question   _____
> 3. wants to check the topic of the question   _____
> 4. wants to check a technical term in the question   _____
> 5. wants to repeat the question to help the audience   _____
> 6. deals with a question that is not related to the study   _____
> 7. wants to give a general answer   _____
> 8. cannot answer   _____
> 9. wants to stop a questioner asking several questions at once   _____
> 10. wants to check if the questioner is satisfied with the answer
>
> 11. wants to show he / she has finished his / her answer   _____
> 12. asks someone to contact him / her later   _____

Script

A
A: I have a question about sintering. How far does it affect the result?
B: Excuse me, what do you mean by sintering?
A: I'm talking about the size of the pores on the ceramic.
B: Okay, I've got you. Well, size is important and, as far as we know, it does affect the quality of the product.

B
A: Could you tell me if this technique can be applied to larger scale production?
B: Actually, we didn't look at that. It wasn't one of the aims of this study.
A: Okay, thank you.

C
A: I think what you are saying is correct. But, I still think the mechanism is different.
B: This is a complicated point. Can we talk about it later?

D
A: I'm interested in the speed at which the reaction took place and also the yield. Could you give me some idea of those two points?
B: Basically, we found that there is a slight increase over time. At the moment, we are still looking at the latest set of data. If you like, I can send you that information when it becomes available.

E
A: I have a question about the catalyst. I'm interested in the speed of the reaction. Could you give me some more information on that?
B: Okay. So this is a question about the catalyst. How fast is the reaction? Well, the answer is, it is a lot faster. And the reason for this is . . .

F
A: My question is about the reaction rate. If we increase the rate by say 5 percent, can we expect the yield to increase accordingly?
B: I'm sorry, I don't follow your question.
A: Okay, I'd like to know about the reaction rate. Does the yield increase?

G

A:I'm interested in the data you showed at the beginning of your presentation about mortality rates. Could you let me have another look at that, please?

B:Okay, just a moment. Are you asking about the data shown in slide 5?

A:Yes, that's right. I want to know why . . .

H

A:You've explained two kinds of treatment. How do patients respond?

B:With either of these kinds of treatments, patients should show considerable improvement. The key is follow up and constant monitoring. Thank you.

I

A:How do these results relate to the results reported last year by researchers at MIT?

B:I'm sorry, I can't answer that. At the moment, I can't give you any definite data.

J

A:Okay, I have a couple of questions. The first one concerns the selection of the parameters for this experiment. The second one is about . . .

B:Can I take your first question now, please?

A:Sure.

K

A:So this represents something of a problem.

B:Yes. What this means is that because different countries have different ways of collecting and calculating trade statistics, comparisons between sets of data are difficult. I hope that answers your question.

L

A:I was interested in what you said about lipids. Could you give me some more information, please?

B:Excuse me, I didn't catch your question.

A:I'm interested in lipids. Could I have some more information on lipids, please?

B:Sure. The main point about lipids is that . . .

Answers

Listening 1 1-l, 2-g, 3-i, 4-j, 5-f, 6-e, 7-b, 8-h, 9-c, 10-d, 11-k, 12-a

Listening 2 1.catch, 2.follow, 3.asking about, 4.mean by, 5.question about, 6.look at, aims, 7.Basically, 8.answer, 9.take, now, 10.hope, answers, 11.Thank you, 12.talk about

Listening 3 1-L, 2-F, 3-G, 4-A, 5-E, 6-B, 7-D, 8-I, 9-J, 10-K, 11-H, 12-C

2 Defining question types

The question and answer session is probably the most difficult part of the presentation to handle, since it is unpredictable and therefore difficult to prepare for. To help presenters, I have classified the main types of questions that occur in the Q and A session. I also provide information on the frequency of these question types. Questions can be divided into five types which I will explain here with examples.

Type 1: More information

Approximately 50 percent of all questions in Q and A sessions are requests for more information about the data presented. This is quite natural as people want information which will help them in their own research.

Here are some examples of questions where the speaker asks for more information.

- *I have a question about the catalyst. How did you select it? And, on what basis?*
- *Could you give me some more information about / on the recycling process?*
- *I was interested in what you said about computer simulation. Could you tell me how long a typical simulation takes?*
- *I'd like to know some of the advantages of your new system.*
- *You didn't mention the role of ligands. Could you give me some more information about / on that?*

Please note that the following sentence is NOT correct.

Please teach me the reaction temperature.

You should change the word *please* to *could you*, and the word *teach* to *tell*.

Could you tell me the reaction temperature, (please)?

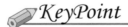KeyPoint

●質疑の 50％は，より詳しい情報を求めるものである．

Type 2: Clarifying information

The second most common type of question is clarifying information. Such questions aim at checking the information that appeared in the presentation. In many cases, the person asking the question wishes to check that his or her understanding of the data is correct. This type of question accounts for more than 20 percent of all questions in the Q and A.

Here are some examples of clarification type questions.

- *I was interested in what you said about the reaction. Did you say that it took place at 20 degrees centigrade?*
- *I'm interested in the period of data collection. Am I right in thinking that the data you showed in slide 7 was collected over a period of just 24 hours?*
- *I have a question about resolution. Did you say that with the new system there is an improvement in resolution of over 10 percent?*
- *Could I just check one point? I think you said that recovery time is 3 or 4 days? Is that right?*
- *I'd like to check one point. Do your trade figures include data for the EU as well?*

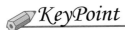 *KeyPoint*

●質疑の 20％は，講演内容についての確認である．

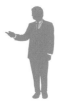

Type 3: Comments

For the presenter, comments are more difficult to handle than the direct questions found in question types 1 and 2. One problem is simply telling the difference between a comment and a direct question. What is the function of a comment? Comments generally offer some explanation for unexplained phenomena described in the presentation, or make comparisons with the questioner's own experience or research. In the Q and A session, comments account for about 15 percent of all the exchanges between the presenter and audience.

Here are some examples.

- *In our data, we found recovery time was about 3 days. This is somewhat different from what you have mentioned today. <u>Could you comment on that, please?</u>*
- *I'm wondering if there is a connection between recovery time and drug selection. <u>Do you have any thoughts on that?</u>*
- *This is more of a comment than a question. If countries have different ways of calculating the data, it seems to me a universal system would be an advantage. <u>What do you think about that?</u>*
- *Can I just comment on the age of onset in patients with this disease? In our data, we found the disease commonly started at around 55 years of age in males. <u>Do you have any comments on that?</u>*
- *This is just a comment. I think the rate of increase shown in Figure 2 suggests other possible causes. <u>How do you feel about that?</u>*
- *<u>I'd like to raise a couple of points.</u> First, the data you have presented excludes some developing countries. And, secondly, there is an obvious need for a centralized system.*
- *<u>I have several observations to make.</u> Firstly, there is the problem of relapse. We also need to consider gum sensitivity and differences between patients. You didn't refer to them in your presentation. <u>Could you comment on these points, please?</u>*

Please do not confuse the following questions.

- *What do you think about that?*
- *How do you feel about that?*

<u>You CANNOT say</u>, How do you think about that? or How do you think about + (topic)?

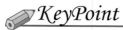

KeyPoint

●質疑の 15%は一般的なコメントで，演者が説明しなかったことについての説明・補足や，演者と質問者の結果の比較などである．

Type 4: Criticism

I often ask presenters to estimate how many questions and comments in the Q and A session involve criticism. Answers vary from less than 5 percent to about 20 percent. In my experience of observing presentations, it's about 10 percent or less. What this means is that only a small proportion of questions and comments are directly critical of the presentation.

I think it is worth considering the function of criticism in the Q and A session. Basically, criticism aims to establish scientific truth; the questioner asks the presenter to explain, confirm, or in some cases, defend his or her experimental methods, results or conclusions. The aim is not to damage the credibility of the presenter or the data, but to establish scientific truth. In this sense, criticism is not necessarily negative. Accordingly, we have to keep in mind that criticism is a normal and important part of the scientific process. When we realize this, criticism becomes less of a threat.

Here are some examples.

- *It seems to me that a different dose would achieve better results.*
- *I was interested in your description of X-ray diffractometry. But I doubt if this method can be applied to very thin films.*
- *How can you be sure that the interaction stops at this point?*
- *I'm sorry, but I don't see how your technique can be applied to samples at higher temperatures.*
- *Are you sure that these data really support your conclusion?*

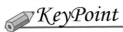 *KeyPoint*

●質疑の 10%弱は科学的根拠を確立するための批評である.

Type 5: Suggestions

Sometimes if a presenter talks about a problem that is unsolved or for which more research is required, people in the audience who have had similar experiences will offer suggestions based on their own experiences.

Here are some examples.

- *Perhaps it would be an idea to recalculate the uncertainty.*
- *Have you tried repeating the experiment under different conditions?*
- *Couldn't you start the experiment at a higher initial temperature?*
- *Why don't you include trade figures for developing countries in your data?*
- *Did you try measuring the waist hip ratio?*

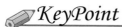

KeyPoint

●質疑には, 不明な部分やさらに研究が必要な部分についての提言もある.

※ p. 101 ～ 103 **Listening 1, 2** の *Answers* は p. 105 に掲載.

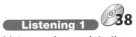

Listen and complete the sentences. Each space has one word.

Type 1: More information

1. _____ _____ _____ _____ some more information about the selection criteria?

2. _____ _____ _____ _____ some more about the experimental setup?

3. _____ _____ _____ _____ _____ the reaction. What was the temperature?

4. _____ _____ _____ _____ uncertainty. What were the causes of uncertainty?

5. _____ _____ _____ _____ the reaction speed. How much faster was it than in the previous method?

Type 2: Clarifying information

1. I'm interested in when the symptoms occurred. _____ _____ _____ _____ the patient had symptoms from the age of 11?

2. _____ _____ _____ _____ _____ that dopamine D5 is reduced in patients with Parkinson's disease?

3. _____ _____ _____ _____ _____? The level of uncertainty in experiment two was the lowest of all the experiments. Is that correct?

4. So patients had one course of postoperative chemotherapy with Cisplatin. _____ _____ _____?

5. _____ _____ data was collected from five locations,_____? How were those locations selected?

Type 3: Comments

1. I _____ _____ _____ _____ to make. First, the reaction time seems faster than usual. Second, I think that using a different catalyst would be useful.

2. I _____ _____ _____ _____ a couple of points.

3. Okay, _____ _____ _____ _____ _____. Under normal circumstances, the initial temperature is usually set at 15 degrees.

4. Just _____ _____ _____ _____. I think you will find that with this drug, the patient will begin to respond to treatment within a few days.

5. _____ _____ _____ _____ one point about the thickness of the films. If you used a thinner film, I think it would improve the results.

Type 4: Criticism

1. You said the temperature increases rapidly and reaches 75 degrees. I find this very _____ _____ _____. In our own experiments, temperature increase never went above 50 degrees.
2. _____ can you _____ the chemical reaction?
3. _____ _____ _____ this can be explained in another way? For example, increased dosage has a negative and not a positive effect.
4. Excuse me, but _____ _____ _____ this method can be applied to experiments at high temperatures.
5. I'm sorry, but _____ _____ _____ that your results match your conclusions.

Type 5: Suggestions

1. _____ _____ _____ _____ changing the weight of the sample?
2. _____ _____ _____ _____ a good idea to take into account the basic differences between the two methods.
3. _____ _____ _____ any alternative treatments?
4. _____ _____ _____ _____ that might solve this problem.
5. _____ _____ _____ measuring the waist hip ratio?

Script
Type 1: More information
1. Could you give me some more information about the selection criteria?
2. Could you tell me some more about the experimental setup?
3. I want to ask about the reaction. What was the temperature?
4. My question is about uncertainty. What were the causes of uncertainty?
5. I have a question about the reaction speed. How much faster was it than in the previous method?

Type 2: Clarifying information
1. I'm interested in when the symptoms occurred. Did you say that the patient had symptoms from the age of 11?
2. Am I right in thinking that dopamine D5 is reduced in patients with Parkinson's disease?
3. Could I check one point? The level of uncertainty in experiment two was the lowest of all the experiments. Is that correct?
4. So patients had one course of postoperative chemotherapy with Cisplatin. Is that right?
5. You said data was collected from five locations, right? How were those locations selected?

Type 3: Comments
1. I have a few observations to make. First, the reaction time seems faster than usual. Second, I think that using a different catalyst would be useful.
2. I would like to raise a couple of points.
3. Okay, this is just a comment. Under normal circumstances, the initial temperature is usually set at 15 degrees.
4. Just a couple of points. I think you will find that with this drug, the patient will begin to respond to treatment within a few days.
5. I'd like to make one point about the thickness of the films. If you used a thinner film, I think it would improve the results.

Type 4: Criticism
1. You said the temperature increases rapidly and reaches 75 degrees. I find this very hard to accept. In our own experiments, temperature increase never went above 50 degrees.
2. How can you explain the chemical reaction?
3. Don't you think this can be explained in another way? For example, increased dosage has a negative and not a positive effect.
4. Excuse me, but I doubt if this method can be applied to experiments at high temperatures.
5. I'm sorry, but I don't think that your results match your conclusions.

Type 5: Suggestions
1. Did you think about changing the weight of the sample?
2. Perhaps it would be a good idea to take into account the basic differences between the two methods.
3. Have you considered any alternative treatments?
4. I have a suggestion that might solve this problem.
5. Have you tried measuring the waist hip ratio?

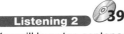 Listening 2 **39**

You will hear ten sentences from a Q & A session. What type of sentences are they? Put the sentences 1~10 into one of the five categories listed below. Each category has two sentence types.

Question Type 1: More information	_____
Question Type 2: Clarification	_____
Question Type 3: Comments	_____
Question Type 4: Criticism	_____
Question Type 5: Suggestions	_____

Script
1. Am I right in thinking that both samples are biodegradable?
2. I was interested in your data from the EU. Could you give me some more information about that?
3. I think your method is useful. But I doubt if it can be used with very thin films.
4. You said that granite can be found in this area. Are there any other interesting rocks in the same area?
5. I have one suggestion to make. Why don't you conduct another experiment at a higher frequency?
6. I have a couple of observations to make. First, the initial temperature seems very low to me. Second, selection of a different catalyst might yield different results.
7. I'd just like to check one point. Did you say that the patients ranged in age between 39 and 47?
8. In my opinion, if you had used a different dose, the results would have been quite different.
9. Have you tried reducing the number of drugs given? I think that would make a difference.
10. In our data, we found recovery time was 3 days, whereas in the data you presented, it was much longer. What's your opinion on that?

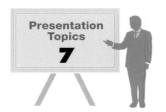

Buzz sessions

Recently, I came across the term buzz session in a conference handbook. In fact, when I looked closely, I found there were several buzz sessions scheduled over the course of the conference, each one lasting an hour. I must admit I had never heard of a buzz session before. Of course, I knew that the word buzz is used to describe the sound of people talking a lot in an excited way. So I guessed that a buzz session is some kind of open discussion.

As I continued to read the conference handbook, I found some information about buzz sessions. They are described in the following way: **Buzz sessions are interactive, moderated discussions of topics of interest to researchers. Problems are discussed and solutions shared by all participants**.

But what does that mean exactly? I think it means that compared to the rigid structure of the oral presentation, *the buzz session is a less formal, freer structure that allows people to exchange opinions more easily. The aim is to find solutions to specific problems*.

The keywords in the description of buzz sessions in the handbook are **interactive, discussions, solutions,** and **shared by all**. *For non-native speakers of English to participate actively in buzz sessions, you need to be able to listen, think and speak in English in real time*. These are goals that we need to set ourselves and move towards. We also need to realize that the conference scene is constantly changing and that it is necessary to keep up with such changes.

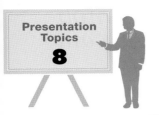

Networking receptions

People who attend conferences regularly will be familiar with the conference banquet, an event usually scheduled on Saturday night which gives everyone the opportunity to relax after a day of presentations. Banquets can be formal, where you have a seat at a table, or less formal where everyone eats and drinks standing up.

The conference scene, however, is changing and in a recent conference program, I noticed that several *networking receptions* were scheduled during the conference. One of the networking receptions was scheduled at exactly the time you would expect a banquet to be scheduled.

I think this suggests a fundamental change in the way people now view social events at conferences. *Whereas previously people attended in order to relax and chat with other participants, now there is a greater emphasis on meeting people in the field, making useful contacts, and exchanging information and ideas.* In some cases, this might lead to job openings, collaborative research and other opportunities.

For researchers who are non-native speakers of English, *networking is just another skill, like that of oral and poster presentations, that has to be learned in order to advance your career.*

Answers (p. 101~103)

Listening 1

Type 1 1.Could you give me, 2.Could you tell me, 3.I want to ask about, 4.My question is about, 5.I have a question about

Type 2 1. Did you say that, 2. Am I right in thinking, 3. Could I check one point, 4. Is that right, 5. You said, right,

Type 3 1. have a few observations, 2. would like to raise, 3. this is just a comment, 4. a couple of points, 5. Id like to make,

Type 4 1. hard to accept, 2. How, explain, 3. Don't you think, 4. I doubt if, 5. I don't think

Type 5 1. Did you think about, 2. Perhaps it would be, 3. Have you considered, 4. I have a suggestion, 5. Have you tried

Listening 2

Type 1—2, 4   Type 2—1, 7   Type 3—6, 10   Type 4—3, 8   Type 5—5 ,9

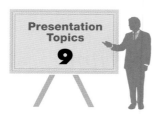

Clarity: How to simplify and rephrase complex information

42

In this section, I would like to look at examples of how presenters aim at clarity by simplifying or rephrasing parts of their presentation that contain complex information.

Here is an example from a presentation.

Notice what happens with adipic acid. The first proton is more like the proton in acetic acid, <u>in other words,</u> the P-K-A has gone up relative to the P-K-A of the succinic acid.

In the above example, the presenter tries to simplify the sentence. The presenter does this by using the phrase *in other words* to introduce a simplified explanation.

In a database of spoken academic English developed at Michigan University, the phrase *in other words* appears 224 times and is the most frequently used phrase when presenters want to simplify what they are saying.

The following verbs are commonly found in phrases used to simplify information: *mean*, *say* and *put*.

Here are some examples:

What I mean is (that) the P-K-A has gone up relative to the P-K-A of the succinic acid.

What I mean to say is (that) the P-K-A has gone up relative to the P-K-A of the succinic acid.

What I'm trying to say is (that) the P-K-A has gone up relative to the P-K-A of the succinic acid.

What I want to say is (that) the P-K-A has gone up relative to the P-K-A of the succinic acid.

To put it another way, the P-K-A has gone up relative to the P-K-A of the succinic acid.

To put it simply, the P-K-A has gone up relative to the P-K-A of the succinic acid.

What about other words and phrases that can be used to simplify and rephrase? For example, *namely*, *that is* and *that is to say*. These words were found to occur infrequently in the database of spoken academic English with frequency rates of less than ten, whereas informal expressions such as, *in other words*, appeared 224 times. This is because *namely*, *that is* and *that is to say* are commonly used in books and academic papers and are too formal for oral presentations.

The problem is that in their presentations many Japanese presenters use *namely*, *that is*, *that is to say* and other formal words and expressions that are more suitable for written English. They prefer the formality of these expressions, but ignore the fact that they are inappropriate for oral presentations. My advice is to use less formal expressions when you want to simplify and re-phrase complex information, such as: *in other words, what I mean is, what I mean to say is, what I'm trying to say is, to put it another way* and *to put it simply*.

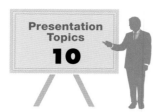

Less is more

In a recent discussion on presentation techniques I was given the following advice: *Less is more*. But, what does 'less is more' really mean? I think it refers to the fact that if we limit the amount of information in our presentation and take care to simplify the material we present, the audience will find it easier to follow than if we present too much data. This means, of course, that we have to carefully edit our presentation, so that what we are presenting is easy for the audience to understand.

This is also true for our slides. Everyone has a tendency to include as much information as possible in their slides. Slides that include too much information are not easy to understand. As a general rule, slides should not have more than 8 lines.

So, when you prepare your next presentation, or even your next slide, you should keep in mind that *less is more*.

【著者略歴】

C.S.Langham

1976 年 ハダースフィールド大学卒業
1982 年 ケント大学大学院修了
2000 年 日本大学歯学部教授（英語）
2020 年 日本大学特任教授

※本書は 2010 年 3 月に「国際学会 English　スピーキング・エクササイズ 口演・発表・応答 音声 CD 付」として発行されたものを，内容は発行時のまま，音声データを CD ではなく，小社 WEB サイトを通じて提供する形式に変更したうえで，再発行したものです．

国際学会 English
スピーキング・エクササイズ
口演・発表・応答
音声 DL 付　　　　　　　　　　　　ISBN978-4-263-43368-3

2023 年 6 月 25 日　第 1 版第 1 刷発行

　　　　　　　　　　　著　者　C. S. Langham
　　　　　　　　　　　発行者　白　石　泰　夫
　　　　　　　発行所　医歯薬出版株式会社
　　　　　〒113-8612　東京都文京区本駒込1−7−10
　　　　　TEL. (03) 5395−7638 (編集)・7630 (販売)
　　　　　FAX. (03) 5395−7639 (編集)・7633 (販売)
　　　　　　　　　　https://www.ishiyaku.co.jp/
　　　　　　　　　　郵便振替番号 00190−5−13816
乱丁，落丁の際はお取り替えいたします　　印刷・あづま堂印刷／製本・愛千製本所

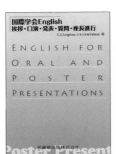
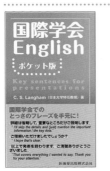